simply
PLANT BASED

fabulous food for a healthy life

Vanita Rahman, MD

Book Publishing Company
SUMMERTOWN, TENNESSEE

Library of Congress Cataloging-in-Publication Data available upon request.

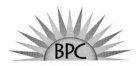

We chose to print this title on responsibly harvested paper stock certified by the Forest Stewardship Council®, an independent auditor of responsible forestry practices. For more information, visit us.fsc.org.

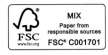

MIX
Paper from
responsible sources
FSC® C001701

Food photography: Asif Rahman
Cover photos: Asif Rahman
Stock photography: 123 RF
Cover and interior design: John Wincek

Printed in China

BPC
PO Box 99
Summertown, TN 38483
888-260-8458
bookpubco.com

ISBN: 978-1-57067-404-4

26 25 24 23 22 21   1 2 3 4 5 6 7 8 9

Disclaimer: The information in this book is presented for educational purposes only. It isn't intended to be a substitute for the medical advice of a physician, dietitian, or other health-care professional.

Contents

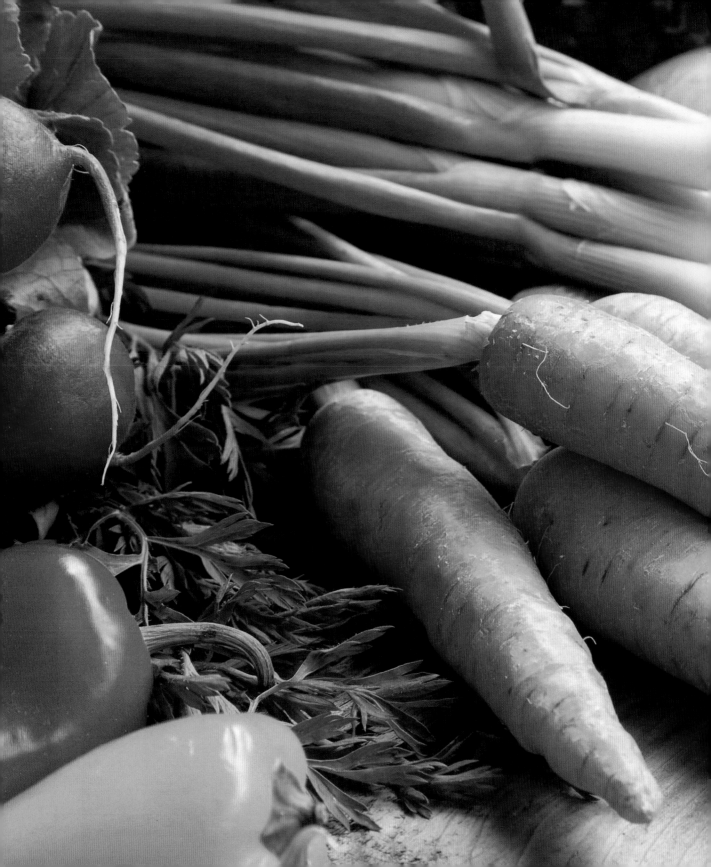

1

Why Eat Plant Based?

You have no doubt heard that a high-quality diet plays a key role in maintaining good health, but what actually constitutes a high-quality diet? With so much conflicting information coming from many different sources—contemporary media, family, friends, colleagues, and even health-care professionals—it can be hard to sort out which foods are health-supporting and which are not. As a practicing physician, clinical researcher, certified nutritionist, and exercise specialist, I am here to clear up the confusion for you. Although any diet can lead to short-term weight loss, only a plant-based diet has been proven to lead to long-term weight loss and improved health.

This is not my opinion or personal preference but what rigorous scientific research has shown—research done at some of the most prestigious medical institutions, such as the Cleveland Clinic and the University of California San Francisco School of Medicine.[1-5] Plant-based diets can lead to lasting weight loss and reverse some of our most common diseases, such as prediabetes and diabetes, high blood pressure, high cholesterol levels, and cardiovascular disease, which is the leading cause of death in the United States and worldwide.[1-13]

If plant-based diets are so beneficial, why aren't more health-care providers recommending them? The reason is that most physicians are not given much instruction about nutrition. Most medical schools offer barely more than nineteen hours of education in the field of nutrition. Nineteen hours of nutrition education may sound significant, but it accounts for less than 1 percent of total lecture time, and most of that is in the form of complex biochemistry rather than practical dietary knowledge.[14-15] If your health-care provider is not talking about the benefits of plant-based diets, that is because they simply do not know about them.

I know this firsthand because I suffered from multiple health problems: excess body weight, prediabetes, high cholesterol levels, arthritis, asthma, allergies, heartburn, and thyroid cancer. Despite the fact that I was a physician, I struggled to manage my multiple health problems. At one point, I was taking more than six medications daily, all of which cost money and had side effects, and none of which targeted the root of the problem. When a medication caused unpleasant side effects, I was prescribed another medication, a process that, to me, as a physician with no nutrition training at the time, seemed normal. Unfortunately, the new medication came with its own set of side effects. It seemed as though my health was spiraling out of control, and I felt lost, scared, and hopeless. I didn't just want to take medications to manage my conditions; I wanted to reverse them. Knowing that I couldn't do that with traditional medications, I looked for alternatives. I explored the connection between nutrition and disease and discovered that the key to good health started at the end of my fork.

Consequently, I began my plant-based journey, and the results exceeded my expectations. I had lost weight many times previously, but I also had always regained it after a few months. This time was different. Not only did I lose the extra weight but I was also able to keep it off. That's because I felt happy and satisfied with the food I was eating. I didn't feel starved or deprived as I had so often before. I liked the food a lot more than I thought I would, and I felt nourished in ways I hadn't experienced in the past. Even more importantly, my health improved: my blood sugar and cholesterol levels normalized; I no longer needed inhalers or antacids; and my joints felt stronger than ever. I had accomplished what I had never imagined was possible: I had reversed my health conditions and regained control of my well-being. And there were some happy surprises along the way. My family was inspired by my successes and joined me in my plant-based journey. My new lifestyle also helped me become a better physician. I fundamentally changed the way I practiced medicine as I integrated diet and lifestyle into patient care. I want to help you achieve the same successes with your health.

You may be eager to improve your health with a plant-based diet and likely have some questions and concerns. Let's tackle a few of the most common ones:

Q: Can I get all the nutrients I need from a plant-based diet?

A: A well-balanced plant-based diet provides all the necessary nutrients except for vitamins B_{12} and D. Vitamin B_{12} is an essential nutrient that our bodies cannot make; we must ingest it via food or supplements. When people consume animal-based foods, they get vitamin B_{12} that was produced by microbes in the gut of the animal. Historically, we got vitamin B_{12} from plants because they contained B_{12} produced by microbes in the soil. Today, however, microbes have vanished from soil due to chemicals used in industrial farming.

For plant-based eaters, it is crucial to consume this vitamin as a supplement. The daily requirement is very small—just over 2 micrograms per day—which can be found in most over-the-counter vitamin B_{12} or B-complex supplements. Although some plant-based foods, such as fortified nutritional yeast and fortified plant-based milks, also contain vitamin B_{12}, they are not reliable sources; there-fore, it is best to take a supplement. Your health-care provider can check your vitamin B_{12} levels to see if they are within the recommended range.

Vitamin D plays a key role in health, and our bodies are designed to produce it in response to sun exposure. However, many people do not have adequate lev-els of vitamin D for a variety of reasons, such as limited access to sunlight. I rec-ommend working with your health-care provider to check your vitamin D levels so you can supplement as needed.

Q: Do plant-based diets provide sufficient protein?

A: First, let's clarify how much protein we need, which is far less than we have been led to believe from mass marketing. Just 10–15 percent of our daily calories should be from protein. Second, as shown in table 1 (below), it is easy to meet this requirement from plants. Unless we are only eating fruits, we will get sufficient protein from a plant-based diet.

TABLE 1. Calories from Protein in Plant-Based Foods

PLANT-BASED FOOD	CALORIES FROM PROTEIN
Legumes (beans, peas, and lentils)	20–50%
Vegetables	10–50%
Whole Grains	10–15%
Fruits	Approximately 5%

Q: I have heard that omega-3 fats found in fish are good for us. How can I get them from a plant-based diet?

A: Omega-3 fats are a type of essential fat we cannot make and must consume in our food. Fish provide two types of omega-3 fats: eicosapentaenoic acid (EPA) and docosahexaenoic acid (DHA). However, fish are also high in cholesterol, fat, and mercury, and they contain no fiber. Plant foods do not contain DHA and EPA but are rich in alpha-linolenic acid (ALA), which our bodies can convert to DHA and EPA. For people age fourteen and up, the daily adequate intake of ALA is 1.1 grams for females and 1.6 grams for males. Women need a little bit more during pregnancy (1.4 grams) and lactation (1.3 grams). As shown in table 2 (below), it is easy to meet our daily requirement of omega-3 fats from plant-based foods. Just 2 teaspoons of flaxseeds or chia seeds or 1 ounce of walnuts per day can provide the necessary amounts.

TABLE 2. Plant-Based Sources of ALA

PLANT-BASED SOURCES OF ALA	ALA CONTENT (GRAMS)
English walnuts (1 ounce)	2.57
Chia seeds (2 teaspoons)	1.69
Flaxseeds (2 teaspoons)	1.57
Black walnuts (1 ounce)	0.76
Edamame (½ cup)	0.28
Vegetarian refried beans (½ cup)	0.21

Q: Is it safe to consume soy products? Will the estrogens in soy increase the risk of breast cancer in women or encourage breast development in boys and men?

A: Whether or not estrogens increase the risk of breast cancer depends on their source and the receptors with which they bind. Certain estrogens, such as the ones produced by our bodies or found in medications, bind with estrogen receptors in the breast that increase the risk of breast cancer. However, the estrogens found in soy products (known as phytoestrogens) bind with a different set of receptors in the breast and decrease the risk of breast-cancer development or recurrence. There is no known evidence that soy products lead to breast development in boys or men.

CHAPTER 1

Q: How do I put together a well-balanced plant-based meal? Will I be limited to eating cold salads? Will the food satisfy me or my family?

A: Learning to prepare plant-based meals is like learning to cook any new cuisine. It may seem overwhelming at first, but with helpful recipes and guidance, such as those found in this book, cooking will become effortless and fun. I share how to easily prepare well-balanced, nutritious, and satisfying meals that you and your family can enjoy. There is a lot more to plant-based meals than a cold salad—unless, of course, that is what you crave. Flip through this book and check out all the recipes for delicious soups, casseroles, pastas, tacos, sandwiches, and desserts!

Q: How will the recipes in this book help me with my health?

A: Not all plant-based foods are healthful. Research has shown that plant-based meals rich in whole-food ingredients and low in fat, sodium, and added sugar lead to healthier outcomes.[17-18] Foods that are high in fat, such as fried foods, can raise blood sugar levels. Foods that are high in sodium, such as processed foods, can raise blood pressure. Foods that are high in saturated fat, such as coconut and palm oil, can raise cholesterol levels. The recipes in this book combine minimally processed ingredients—fruits, vegetables, whole grains, legumes, herbs, and spices—to create meals that are low in fat, sugar, and sodium and high in fiber and nutrients. If you are looking to lose weight; lower your blood sugar, blood pressure, or cholesterol; improve joint pain; increase your energy; or gain control over your health, then this is the cookbook for you.

Q: How can I sustain this way of eating long-term?

A: Plant-based eating is not a fad diet nor a short-term solution; it is a lifestyle. In order to sustain this lifestyle long-term, the food has to be tasty, because if it isn't enjoyable, the lifestyle won't be sustainable. I spent years curating the recipes in this book to make them nutritious, flavorful, and easy to prepare. They have been vetted by a growing family with diverse tastes and even some picky eaters. Now it's your turn to enjoy these delicious dishes.

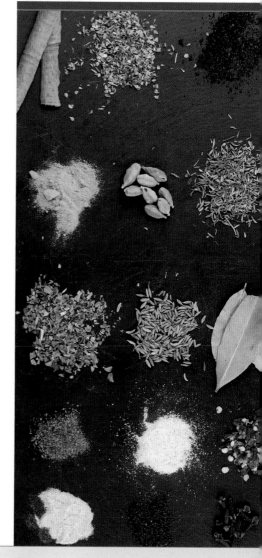

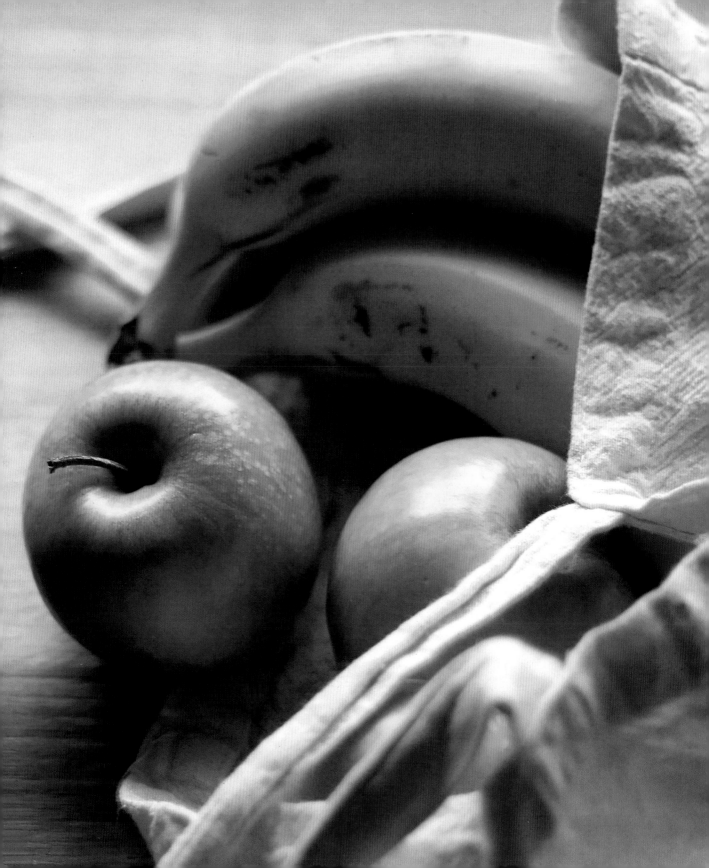

2

Grocery Shopping and Meal Planning

At this point, you are ready to start your plant-based lifestyle, but you may be wondering how to begin. No worries—this chapter has you covered. The key to a successful transition is planning ahead and stocking your kitchen with essential items. In this chapter, we will put together a grocery list and a weekly meal plan to help you get started.

Tips for Grocery Shopping

A trip to the grocery store can be fun or onerous depending on your mood, the time of day, and your other responsibilities. But a well-planned grocery list and helpful suggestions can make the experience go much more smoothly. Here are some tips to bear in mind before you head out to the store:

AVOID SHOPPING WHEN YOU'RE HUNGRY. Have you ever gone grocery shopping when you're hungry? What was it like? Hunger is a powerful emotion that makes it much more difficult to stick with healthy choices. It is also easy to buy too much when you're hungry. Having a small snack or meal before you head to the grocery store can help you stay on track.

KEEP A RUNNING GROCERY LIST. Have you ever returned from the grocery store and realized that you're missing a key ingredient for the recipe you had in mind or that you purchased something you already had in the house? A grocery list can

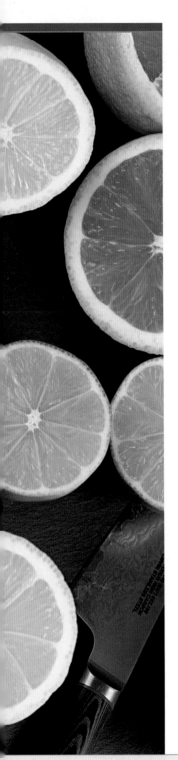

help you avoid these common pitfalls. Use your smartphone, a pocket diary, or even a folded piece of paper to jot down grocery items as you think of them. Also, check your pantry and refrigerator before you head out to see if the items are already in your kitchen.

GET TO KNOW YOUR NEIGHBORHOOD GROCERY STORES. No single store is likely to carry everything you need. Different stores carry different items, and even the same items may range in price among them. As you shop your local stores, you will develop a sense of what each one offers, including bargains.

MINIMIZE THE USE OF PROCESSED FOODS. As much as possible, stick with unprocessed foods, such as fresh fruits, vegetables, dried beans, and whole grains. Avoid processed foods, which includes anything that is premade, such as canned foods (other than beans), sauces, dressings, and frozen meals. These items tend to be high in added fats, sugar, sodium, and calories.

Basic Pantry and Refrigerator Items

As you stock your kitchen, it is helpful to think of food items in eight general groups: fruits, vegetables, legumes (beans, peas, and lentils), grains, herbs and spices, condiments, vegan milks, and nuts and seeds. Table 1 (page 3) lists the staple items in each group. Let's take a look at each group in more detail.

FRUITS

Fruits are nature's perfect ready-to-eat snack and an important part of a healthy diet. People with diabetes are sometimes concerned about the amount of sugar in fruits. However, it is important to appreciate that, while fruits do contain a small amount of natural sugar, it is insignificant compared to the added sugars in desserts such as cookies and ice cream. Additionally, the sugar in fruits is bundled with important nutrients, including fiber, vitamins, and minerals. For example, fruits are high in potassium, which helps lower blood pressure levels, and most Americans do not consume sufficient amounts of potassium. Aim for three to five servings of fresh fruits daily. One serving is equivalent to one-half cup of berries or chopped fruit or one small apple or banana. Some fruits are available year-round while others are seasonal, such as mangoes, peaches, and pomegranates.

Frozen fruits are just as nutritious as fresh ones, but avoid canned fruits because they are usually processed with added sugars and syrups. It is also important to avoid fruit juices, which are concentrates of the sugar and water found in fruits, without the beneficial fiber and nutrients. If you are trying to lose weight or lower your blood sugar, it may be best to avoid dried fruits. Fresh fruits are 90 percent water by volume, and dried fruits are produced by removing the water (hence the name "dried fruits"). Dried fruits contain the same amount of sugar and calories as fresh fruits but in one-tenth the volume. And some dried fruits, such as cranberries and pineapple, may contain added sugar. As a result, their caloric density is quite high even though they are fat-free.

TIP: If you have leftover fruits, slice and freeze them. They can be used at a later time for baking or making smoothies and vegan ice creams (see pages 131–132).

VEGETABLES

Just like fruits, vegetables are packed with fiber, potassium, and other essential nutrients. Aim for three to five servings of vegetables daily; a serving size is approximately one-half cup of uncooked vegetables. Enjoy your veggies raw, steamed, roasted, or boiled. Avoid high-fat preparation methods, such as deep-frying or using heavy creams or sauces. It is most important to consume a wide variety of vegetables (for example, leafy greens, broccoli, and cauliflower) on a regular basis. Frozen or fresh vegetables are equally nutritious. However, canned veggies can be high in sodium. There is often concern about the nutrition profile of starchy vegetables, such as white potatoes and sweet potatoes. Potatoes themselves are nutritious; what makes them unhealthy is frying them or consuming

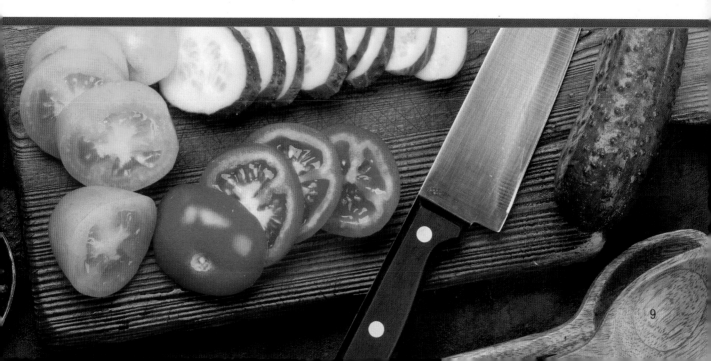

Cooking Beans and Lentils

Beans and lentils are used commonly in plant-based recipes. You can either cook dried beans and lentils or buy canned ones. The idea of cooking dried legumes may seem overwhelming, but it is actually quite simple. The cooking times of various beans and lentils vary, depending on the type of legume and its age, density, and size. Presoaking legumes for 8 to 12 hours will decrease the time needed to boil them. Some lentils cook within minutes and do not require presoaking, while others need to boil for more than an hour after presoaking. For example, orange and red lentils cook within 10 minutes without presoaking. However, it is best to soak dried black beans and chickpeas for 8 to 12 hours, drain and rinse them, cover with fresh water to one inch above the beans, and boil them until soft, 45 to 60 minutes. (Older beans may take substantially longer and may require additional water during cooking.) An alternative to stove-top cooking is using a slow cooker or an electric pressure cooker. The advantage of using these is that you don't have to actively manage the legumes while they are cooking. Note that the size of cooked legumes will be larger than the size of the dried legumes. As a general rule of thumb, legumes usually double in size when they are cooked. Also, know that beans freeze beautifully, so you can cook a large batch, use just what you need, and freeze the remainder.

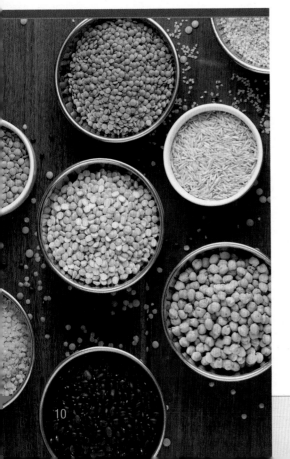

them with high-fat condiments, such as butter, cheese, or cream. Enjoy baked, cooked, or roasted potatoes, and avoid peeling them because the skin contains valuable nutrients. As a bonus, not peeling potatoes also reduces your work.

LEGUMES

Lentils and beans, collectively referred to as legumes, are powerhouses of protein that make for hearty dishes that help us feel full for hours. For example, about 30 percent of the calories in black beans and chickpeas are from protein, and that number jumps to more than 40 percent for tofu and edamame. It is helpful to keep your pantry stocked with dried black beans, chickpeas, and lentils because they have a long shelf life and are excellent replacements for meat, poultry, and fish.

Certain beans and legumes, such as black beans and chickpeas, are readily available canned. When purchasing canned legumes, it is best to select unsalted ones, as those with added salt tend to be high in sodium. If you are unable to

Choosing the Best Flour

ost commercial baked goods are prepared with all-purpose flour, which is refined from whole wheat flour derived from ground red wheat berries. In this book, many of the recipes call for whole wheat pastry flour (also known as white whole wheat flour), which is a whole-grain flour made from naturally white whole wheat berries. It tends to be smoother and milder than standard whole wheat flour. However, if you are unable to find whole wheat pastry flour, you may substitute standard whole wheat flour instead.

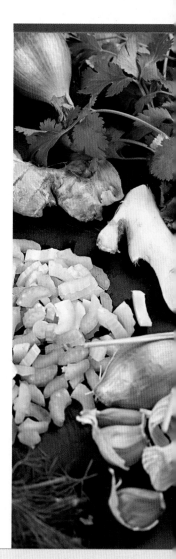

find unsalted varieties, you can rinse the beans well with water and drain them prior to using them in recipes, as rinsing will help remove some of the sodium.

GRAINS

Grains have been unfairly vilified by trendy fad diets, such as low-carb and keto. However, grains are a nutritious and essential part of a well-balanced diet. The key is to stick with whole grains (such as brown rice, oats, quinoa, whole wheat products) rather than refined grains (such as white bread, refined flour, refined pasta, white rice). Whole grains are rich in fiber, vitamins, and minerals and help us feel satiated. The recipes in this book generally use whole grains, and it is helpful to stock a variety of them. They have a long shelf life and stay fresh for months.

HERBS AND SPICES

The recipes in this book use herbs and spices to season foods rather than added fat or sugar. Not only do herbs and spices impart enticing flavor, but they also contain important antioxidants that help our bodies fight inflammation. For example, turmeric is a traditional herb that has been used in various ethnic cuisines for centuries; it gives food a beautiful yellow color and contains natural antioxidants. Stock your kitchen with a variety of dried herbs and spices so they will always be readily available. Table 3 (page 12) lists some of the most useful ones to keep on hand.

CONDIMENTS

This category includes a wide variety of items, such as vinegars, unsweetened cocoa powder, and vanilla extract, that are helpful for flavoring a broad range of

TABLE 3. Sample Grocery List

FOOD GROUP	STAPLE ITEMS		SEASONAL OR RECIPE-BASED ITEMS
CONDIMENTS AND OTHER KITCHEN STAPLES	Balsamic vinegar Canola oil spray Cocoa powder (not Dutch processed), unsweetened Ketchup Red wine vinegar	Sherry vinegar Soy sauce Sriracha sauce Vanilla extract White wine vinegar	
FRUITS	Apples Bananas Berries Grapes		Mangoes Oranges Pears Pomegranates
GRAINS	Brown rice Rolled oats Whole wheat flour or whole wheat pastry flour Whole wheat pasta		Bulgur Lasagna noodles, whole wheat Tortillas, corn or whole wheat
HERBS AND SPICES	Black pepper, ground Cayenne Chipotle chile powder Cinnamon, ground Cumin seeds	Garlic, fresh and granules Italian seasoning Salt Turmeric, ground	Cardamom, ground Cilantro, fresh Oregano, dried Parsley, fresh Smoked paprika
LEGUMES	Black beans, dried or unsalted canned Chickpeas, dried or unsalted canned Red lentils, dried		Edamame, frozen shelled Green lentils, dried Split peas, dried Tofu, firm, extra-firm, and silken Yellow split peas, dried
VEGAN MILKS	Almond, unsweetened plain Soy, unsweetened plain		
VEGETABLES	Avocado Baby carrots Corn, frozen kernels Onions Peas, frozen	Potatoes, red or white Salad greens Sweet potatoes Tomatoes	Artichoke hearts, frozen Broccoli Cauliflower Celery Kale Spinach

dishes. Most items in this category have a long shelf life and keep well for weeks to months. Some of them, such as ketchup and sriracha sauce, are processed foods that can be high in sodium or sugar and are therefore used sparingly in this book.

VEGAN MILKS

It is helpful to stock your kitchen with one or two vegan milks. Although it is not necessary to drink milk (dairy or nondairy) from a health perspective, plant-based milks are enjoyable with cereals and in hot beverages and are useful for adding to recipes. There are many different varieties available; the most popular ones are soy or almond based. Experiment with various types and brands to discover which ones you most prefer.

TIP: Opt for vegan milks without added sugar or oil, and keep in mind that different varieties may work better with certain foods or beverages. For example, some people prefer soy milk with tea or coffee but would rather have almond or flax milk with cereal.

NUTS AND SEEDS

Nuts and seeds have a long shelf life, are ready to eat, and are widely available. However, it is important to appreciate a few characteristics about this group: Nuts and seeds are high in fat; generally, over 70 percent of the calories are from fat. As a result, they have a high caloric density. So, if you are trying to lose weight or lower

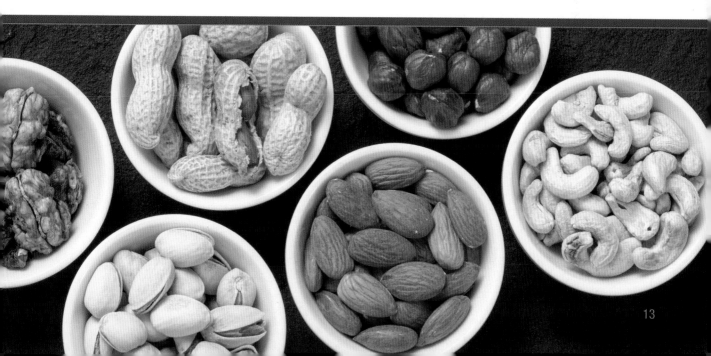

your blood sugar, use nuts and seeds sparingly because they can lead to weight gain and can raise blood sugar levels. They are used minimally in the recipes in this book.

Tips for Meal Planning

Transitioning to a low-fat, plant-based diet can seem overwhelming at first. But with practice and patience, you will soon enjoy spectacular whole-foods meals and reap the tremendous health benefits. Here are some tips to help you get started:

- **Plan a weekly menu.** Flip through this book and select the recipes that appeal to you. Jot them down on a piece of paper; this will help you with grocery shopping and meal preparation. Table 4 (below) provides a sample weekly menu with recipes selected from the book.

- **Prep for the week's meals over the weekend.** For example, the batter for waffles and pancakes can be prepared in advance, which will save precious time during busy mornings. Presoaking and boiling legumes over the weekend will save significant time and effort on active weekdays.

- **Chop vegetables shortly after you purchase them.** Doing this increases the likelihood that you will cook with them. Certain vegetables, such as broccoli, carrots, cauliflower, and kale, are particularly amenable to prechopping because

TABLE 4. Sample Weekly Menu

	BREAKFAST	LUNCH	DINNER
MON	Savory Kale Scones, page 25	Chickpea Tuna Salad Sandwiches, page 93	Veggie Lasagna, page 115
TUE	Whole-Grain Waffles, page 32	Veggie Chili, page 60	Brown Rice Vegetable Pilaf, page 118
WED	Crunchy Granola, page 21	Hummus Sandwiches, page 97	Cauliflower Wings, page 116
THU	Blueberry Muffins, page 26	Minestrone, page 62	Black Bean Tacos, page 124
FRI	No-Cook Muesli, page 22	Avocado Toast with Delicata Squash, page 96	Pasta with No-Cheese Alfredo Sauce, page 75
SAT	Scrambled Tofu, page 36	Falafel Pita Pockets, page 90	Soba Noodles with Vegetables, page 104
SUN	Buckwheat Pancakes, page 31	Yellow Split Pea Veggie Burgers, page 87	Marinated Tofu Steaks, page 107

TABLE 5. Easy Snack Ideas

	SNACK IDEAS		TIPS
FRESH AND FROZEN FRUITS	All fresh fruits and berries Frozen grapes		
GRAINS	Rolled oats		Rolled oats cook within minutes in the microwave or on the stove top and pair well with vegan milk and fresh berries.
LEGUMES	Frozen edamame		Frozen edamame steams within minutes and is a satisfying snack.
NUTS, SEEDS, AND DRIED FRUITS	Assorted nuts, seeds, and dried fruits		These are convenient and filling, but because of their high-fat content and caloric density, they can raise blood sugar and can lead to weight gain.
VEGETABLES	Baby carrots Celery sticks Cherry or grape tomatoes	Cucumber sticks Sweet potato wedges	Baked sweet potatoes make a hearty snack.

they don't release water or discolor afterward. For others, such as onions, potatoes, and tomatoes, it is best to prep them just before cooking because they don't retain their texture or color after they have been chopped.

- **Cook meals for the coming week on the weekend.** This will minimize your effort after a long day at work. Many recipes—such as dips, dressings, grains (bulgur, pasta, quinoa, rice), sauces, scones, and soups—can be prepared ahead of time and will keep well.

- **Cook large portions and freeze the extras.** For example, double a soup recipe and freeze extra portions in single-serving containers. This way you will have a healthy homemade meal whenever you need it.

- **Have some backup meals ready to go.** Keep your kitchen stocked with ingredients for a few easy meals that you can whip up in a hurry. For example, rolled oats and Scrambled Tofu (page 36) take just a few minutes to cook and can be enjoyed for breakfast, lunch, or dinner. Quick and Easy Lentil Soup (page 69) can be prepared within 15 minutes and makes enough for several hearty meals.

- **Be patient with yourself and have fun.** Try a new veggie, herb, or spice. Soon you will become adept at making superb vegan meals and will know your go-to favorites.

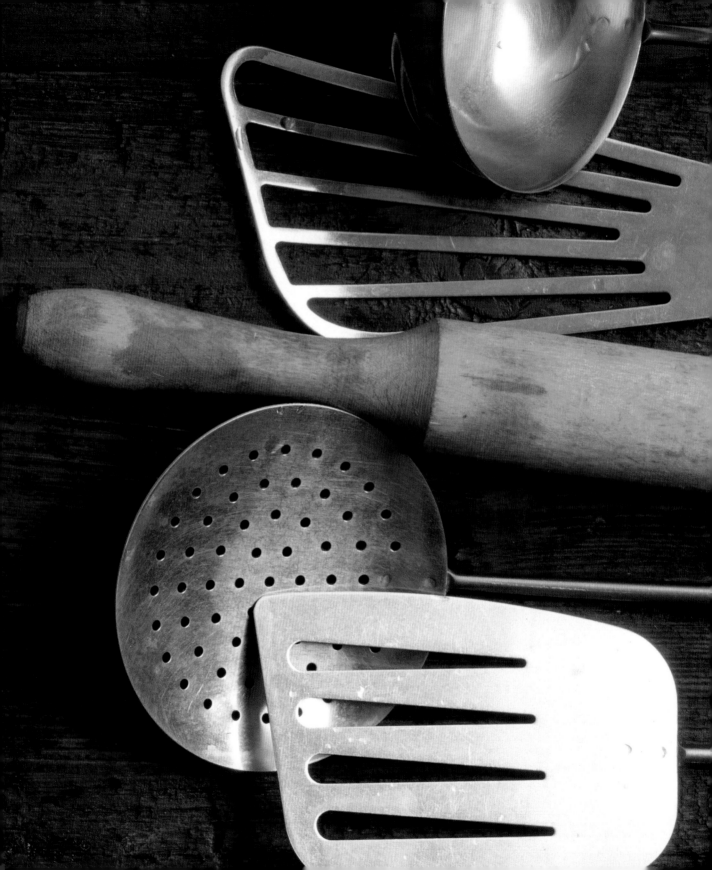

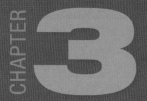

Kitchen Tools and Gadgets That Work for You

n this chapter, I will review various kitchen tools and gadgets that are helpful in day-to-day cooking, can save you time and effort in the kitchen, and can even add some health benefits to your diet. Some of these are relatively simple, nonelectric gadgets, while others are more sophisticated electric appliances.

Nonelectric Kitchen Gadgets

ere's a list of simple kitchen tools that can help decrease your time and workload in the kitchen:

- **Bread knife.** A bread knife is usually long and has a serrated edge that grips and slices the bread easily. It is also very useful for slicing pita rounds and tortillas.

- **Cutting board.** A wooden cutting board with grippy rubber feet works best, as the wooden surface won't dull knives, and the rubber feet will prevent the board from slipping.

- **Garlic press.** It is much easier and faster to crush garlic cloves with a press than to chop them finely with a knife. Crushed garlic also has a smoother taste and texture than chopped garlic.

- **Grater.** This simple tool is very helpful for shredding fruits and vegetables, such as cucumbers, carrots, and potatoes. A small, very fine grater is ideal for grating fresh ginger.

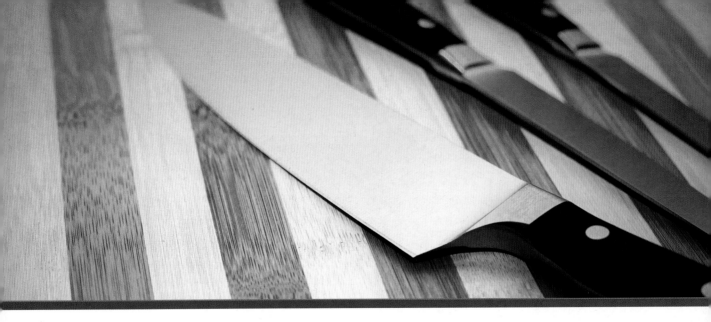

- **Sharp knife.** A sharp knife is very useful for chopping vegetables and fruits, and it reduces the risk of injury because it is less likely to slip. Select the size and style (serrated or smooth) that feels most comfortable to you. Avoid washing cutting knives in the dishwasher because doing so will dull the blade.

- **Lemon press.** A lemon press minimizes the effort required to squeeze lemon or lime juice and simultaneously strains the seeds. You can store excess juice in the refrigerator or freezer for future use.

- **Vegetable peeler.** With a vegetable peeler, the process of peeling fruits and vegetables is almost effortless, especially when compared to using a knife.

Electric Appliances

These appliances can significantly decrease cooking time and effort while also offering health benefits:

- **Air fryer.** An air fryer is a small oven that uses convection heat so that food cooks quickly and has a crispy texture. Traditional deep-fried food is very high in fat, which can lead to weight gain and raise blood sugar levels. But with an air fryer, you can enjoy the taste of crispy food, such as potato fries, Baked Veggie Pakoras (page 121), Marinated Tofu Steaks (page 107), and Cauliflower Wings (page 116), without using any oil.

- **Bread machine.** Most commercially prepared breads are high in sodium, which can raise blood pressure, and they typically are made with refined rather than whole grains. A bread machine allows you to make soft, fluffy, whole-grain breads while limiting the amount of sodium they contain. It takes just a few minutes to put the ingredients into the machine, and then the machine mixes and kneads the dough and bakes the bread without any effort on your part.

- **Electric hand or stand mixer.** Electric hand mixers and stand mixers are useful for preparing batters for baked goods. Stand mixers are much more powerful but also cost significantly more and require more counter space.

- **Electric pressure cooker or slow cooker.** Electric pressure cookers cook food under very high pressure and are therefore able to cook it very quickly. They are particularly useful for cooking dense foods, such as dried beans and legumes. They also cook without the need for frequent monitoring, unlike stove-top cooking. For example, an electric pressure cooker can cook dried black beans or chickpeas within 45 minutes and without any presoaking of the beans. The same task done on the stove top would entail 8 to 12 hours of presoaking followed by 45 minutes or longer of stove-top boiling with frequent monitoring. Electric slow cookers also don't require monitoring. However, they do take much longer to cook the food than electric pressure cookers.

- **Electric rice cooker.** Electric rice cookers are very useful for cooking grains, such as plain rice or rice pilaf, steel-cut oats, and bulgur. They save time because you don't have to tend to the food as it cooks. Some rice cookers also have timers that can be set to cook the food at particular times.

- **Electric waffle iron.** An electric waffle iron cooks the waffle for you, so you don't have to constantly monitor it, which frees up your time to tend to other tasks. If you prepare the batter for Whole-Grain Waffles (page 32) in advance, you can easily dish up nutritious waffles in the morning, especially when you use an electric waffle iron to cook them.

- **High-speed blender or food processor.** High-speed blenders are able to process food at a very high speed. As a result, they can mix dips, dressings, and sauces within minutes, whereas a traditional blender will require much more time and effort. High-speed blenders can also process frozen fruits and vegan milks into smooth ice creams, and these homemade versions are much healthier than commercial ones, which are typically high in added sugar and fat. A food processor can do some of the same tasks as a high-speed blender, but the results may not be as smooth, especially when it comes to blending frozen fruits. However, a food processor offers the added benefit of being able to shred and chop vegetables.

Whole-Grain Waffles

CRUNCHY Granola

Although this nourishing granola is low in added fat and sugar, the taste is irresistible. Serve it with vegan milk or yogurt.

8 cups **rolled oats**

½ cup slivered **almonds**

½ cup crushed **walnuts**

½ cup **raisins**

½ cup **canola** or **vegetable oil**

¼ cup **brown sugar**

¼ cup **maple syrup**

¼ cup **agave nectar**

1 tablespoon **vanilla extract**

1 tablespoon **ground cinnamon**

1. Preheat the oven to 300 degrees F. Line two 13 x 9-inch baking sheets with parchment paper. Alternatively, use nonstick baking sheets.

2. Put the oats, almonds, walnuts, and raisins in a large bowl and stir to combine.

3. Put the oil, sugar, maple syrup, agave nectar, vanilla extract, and cinnamon in a small saucepan and stir to combine. Cook, stirring constantly, over medium-high heat until the mixture comes to a boil. Remove from the heat.

4. Pour the wet ingredients over the dry ingredients and stir until well combined.

5. Divide the mixture evenly between the two baking sheets, spreading it out as thinly as possible.

6. Bake for about 20 minutes, until the oats are golden brown but still a bit moist. Let cool for 20 minutes before serving.

Cool completely before storing. Stored in an airtight container at room temperature, the granola will keep for about 1 week.

No-Cook MUESLI

Rolled oats and fresh fruits are the foundation of this famous Swiss dish. As this version is nut-free, it makes a terrific light morning meal or midday snack.

3 cups whole **berries** (blackberries, blueberries, or raspberries) **or finely chopped strawberries** or **apples**

2½ cups unsweetened plain **soy** or **almond milk**

1½ cups **rolled oats**

2 tablespoons **maple syrup**

Stored in an airtight container in the refrigerator, the muesli will keep for about 3 days.

1 Put all the ingredients in a large bowl and stir until well combined.

2 Cover and refrigerate for at least 8 hours before serving.

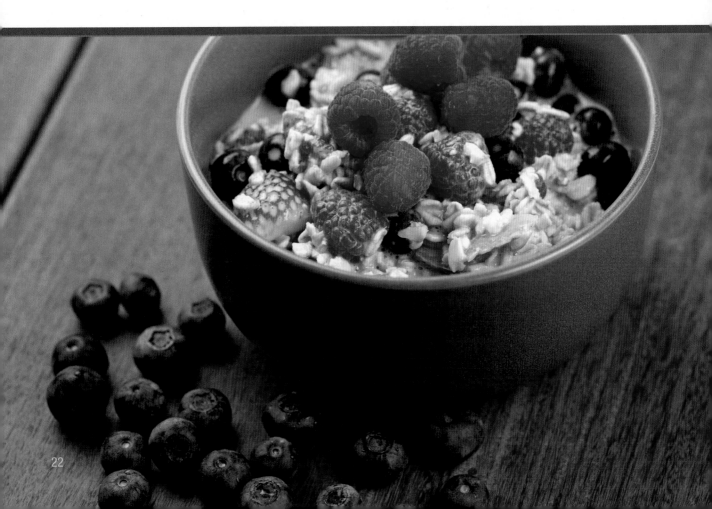

Apricot and Chocolate Chip SCONES

MAKES 12 SCONES

Apricots give these scones a zesty tang, while chocolate chips add sublime appeal. Served with hot tea or coffee, they are stupendous for breakfast or an afternoon snack.

3 cups **whole wheat pastry flour**

¾ cup finely chopped **dried apricots**

½ cup **sugar**

½ cup **vegan chocolate chips**

1 teaspoon **baking powder**

1 cup unsweetened plain **soy** or **almond milk**

¼ cup **olive oil**

1. Preheat the oven to 400 degrees F. Line a large baking sheet with parchment paper.

2. Put the flour, apricots, sugar, chocolate chips, and baking powder in a large bowl and stir until well combined.

3. Add the milk and oil and incorporate using an electric hand or stand mixer until well combined.

4. Using your hands, divide the dough into 12 dollops (about ¼ cup each) and drop them on the lined baking sheet about 2 inches apart. Flatten each dollop slightly with the back of a spoon.

5. Bake for about 20 minutes, until the scones are golden brown and a toothpick inserted into the center of one comes out clean. Let cool on a rack for 5 minutes before serving.

Cool completely before storing. Stored in an airtight container in the refrigerator, the scones will keep for about 4 days. Before serving, warm leftover scones for 5 minutes in the oven preheated to 375 degrees F.

CRANBERRY AND THYME Scones

These whole-grain scones are slightly sweet and slightly savory. They are bursting with cranberry goodness and just a hint of thyme. Serve them with jam and hot tea or coffee.

3 cups **whole wheat pastry flour**

¾ cup **dried cranberries**

½ cup **sugar**

1 teaspoon **baking powder**

1 teaspoon **dried thyme**

½ teaspoon **salt**

1 cup unsweetened plain **soy** or **almond milk**

¼ cup **olive oil**

1 Preheat the oven to 400 degrees F. Line a large baking sheet with parchment paper.

2 Put the flour, cranberries, sugar, baking powder, thyme, and salt in a large bowl and stir until well combined.

3 Add the milk and oil and incorporate using an electric hand or stand mixer until well combined.

4 Using your hands, divide the dough into 12 dollops (about ¼ cup each) and drop them on the lined baking sheet about 2 inches apart. Flatten each dollop slightly with the back of a spoon.

5 Bake for about 20 minutes, until the scones are golden brown and a toothpick inserted into the center of one comes out clean. Let cool on a rack for 5 minutes before serving.

Cool completely before storing. Stored in an airtight container in the refrigerator, the scones will keep for about 4 days. Before serving, warm leftover scones for 5 minutes in the oven preheated to 375 degrees F.

Savory **KALE SCONES**

MAKES 12 SCONES

Kale gives these appetizing scones a pleasant crunch and adds important nutrients, including calcium. What a delicious way to sneak in a few veggies at breakfast!

3 cups **whole wheat pastry flour**

1 teaspoon **baking powder**

¾ teaspoon **salt**

3 cups finely chopped **curly kale,** firmly packed

1 cup unsweetened plain **soy** or **almond milk**

¼ cup **olive oil**

1. Preheat the oven to 400 degrees F. Line a large baking sheet with parchment paper.

2. Put the flour, baking powder, and salt in a large bowl and stir until well combined.

3. Add the kale, milk, and oil and incorporate using an electric hand or stand mixer until well combined.

4. Using your hands, divide the dough into 12 dollops (about ¼ cup each) and drop them on the baking sheet about 2 inches apart. Flatten each dollop slightly with the back of a spoon.

5. Bake for about 20 minutes, until the scones are golden brown and a toothpick inserted into the center of one comes out clean. Let cool on a rack for 5 minutes before serving.

Cool completely before storing. Stored in an airtight container in the refrigerator, the scones will keep for about 4 days. Before serving, warm leftover scones for 5 minutes in the oven preheated to 375 degrees F.

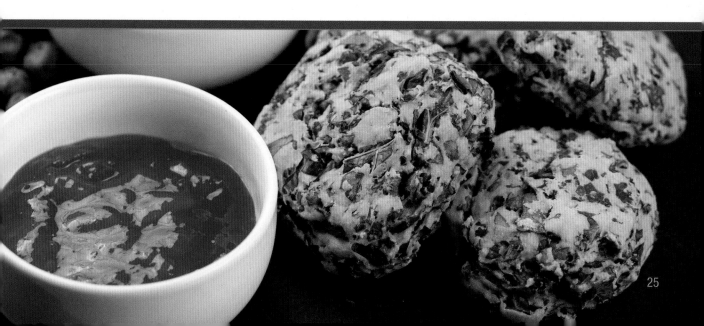

25

BLUEBERRY Muffins

These perennial favorites are made with whole-grain wheat and oat flours and are studded with naturally sweet fresh blueberries.

2 cups **whole wheat pastry flour**

⅔ cup plus 1 tablespoon **sugar**

1 teaspoon **baking powder**

1½ cups unsweetened plain **soy** or **almond milk**

¼ cup **canola** or **vegetable oil**

1 teaspoon **vanilla extract**

2 cups fresh **blueberries**

1. Preheat the oven to 375 degrees F. Line a 12-cup standard muffin pan with cupcake liners.

2. Put the pastry flour, ⅔ cup of the sugar, and the baking powder in a large bowl and stir until well combined.

3. Add the milk, oil, and vanilla extract and incorporate using an electric hand or stand mixer until well combined.

4. Add the blueberries and gently stir until evenly distributed.

5. Spoon evenly into the lined muffin cups. Sprinkle the remaining tablespoon of sugar evenly over the top of the muffins.

6. Bake for about 18 minutes, until a toothpick inserted into the center of a muffin comes out clean. Let cool for 10 minutes before serving.

TIP

Let cool completely before storing. Stored in an airtight container in the refrigerator, the muffins will keep for about 4 days.

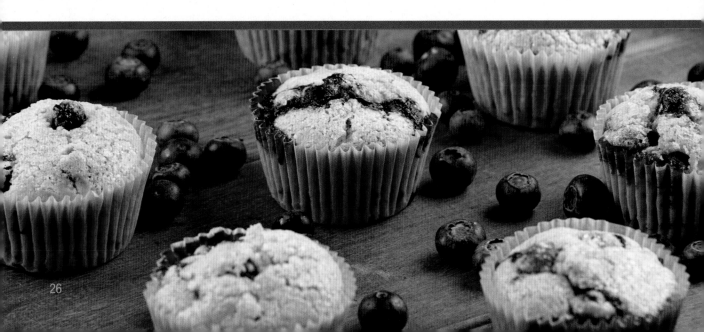

Lemon MUFFINS

These whole-grain muffins are enlivened with fresh lemon zest and juice for a wonderful sweet-tart taste.

2 cups **whole wheat pastry flour**

1½ teaspoons **baking powder**

Zest of 1 **lemon** (about 1 tablespoon)

⅛ teaspoon **salt**

1 cup unsweetened plain **soy** or **almond milk**

½ cup **maple syrup**

⅓ cup **olive oil**

¼ cup freshly squeezed **lemon juice**

1. Preheat the oven to 350 degrees F. Line a 12-cup standard muffin pan with cupcake liners.

2. Put the flour, baking powder, lemon zest, and salt in a large bowl and stir until well combined.

3. Put the milk, maple syrup, and oil in a medium bowl and stir until well combined.

4. Pour the wet ingredients into the dry ingredients and incorporate using an electric hand or stand mixer until well combined.

5. Add the lemon juice and stir until well incorporated.

6. Spoon evenly into the lined muffin cups.

7. Bake for about 25 minutes, until a toothpick inserted into the center of a muffin comes out clean. Let cool for 10 minutes before serving.

Let cool completely before storing. Stored in an airtight container in the refrigerator, the muffins will keep for about 4 days.

Pumpkin **BREAD**

This seasonal delicacy is moist and fragrant with sweet spices. It's especially welcome on chilly autumn mornings.

1¾ cups **whole wheat pastry flour**

½ cup **brown sugar**

1 teaspoon **baking soda**

1 teaspoon **ground cinnamon**

½ teaspoon **salt**

½ teaspoon **baking powder**

½ teaspoon **ground nutmeg**

½ teaspoon **ground ginger**

1 (15-ounce) can unsweetened **pumpkin purée**

¼ cup smooth **almond butter**

¼ cup unsweetened **applesauce**

2 tablespoons **water**

2 tablespoons **maple syrup**

1 tablespoon raw **pumpkin seeds**

1½ teaspoons **sugar** (preferably coarse sugar with large crystals)

1. Preheat the oven to 350 degrees F. Line a 9 x 5-inch loaf pan with parchment paper.

2. Put the flour, brown sugar, baking soda, cinnamon, salt, baking powder, nutmeg, and ginger in a large bowl and stir until well combined.

3. Add the pumpkin purée, almond butter, applesauce, water, and maple syrup and incorporate using an electric hand or stand mixer until well combined.

4. Pour into the lined loaf pan. Sprinkle the pumpkin seeds and sugar evenly over the top.

5. Bake for about 50 minutes, until a toothpick inserted into the center comes out clean. Let cool for 10 minutes before slicing.

Cool completely before storing. Stored in an airtight container in the refrigerator, the bread will keep for about 4 days.

CHOCOLATE Banana Bread

MAKES 6 SERVINGS

hocolate chips, bananas, and pecans team up in this moist, quick bread that appeals to children, teens, and adults alike.

1 cup **whole wheat pastry flour**

1 cup **oat flour**

⅔ cup **sugar**

⅓ cup **vegan chocolate chips**

1 teaspoon **baking soda**

¼ teaspoon **salt**

2 very ripe large **bananas,** mashed

½ cup unsweetened plain **soy** or **almond milk**

¼ cup smooth **almond butter**

¼ cup unsweetened **applesauce**

2 tablespoons crushed **pecans**

1 Preheat the oven to 350 degrees F. Line a 9 x 5-inch loaf pan with parchment paper.

2 Put the pastry flour, oat flour, sugar, chocolate chips, baking soda, and salt in a large bowl and stir until well combined.

3 Add the bananas, milk, almond butter, and applesauce and incorporate using an electric hand or stand mixer until well combined.

4 Pour into the lined loaf pan. Sprinkle the pecans evenly over the top.

5 Bake for about 45 minutes, until a toothpick inserted into the center comes out clean. Let cool for 10 minutes before slicing.

Cool completely before storing. Stored in an airtight container in the refrigerator, the bread will keep for about 4 days.

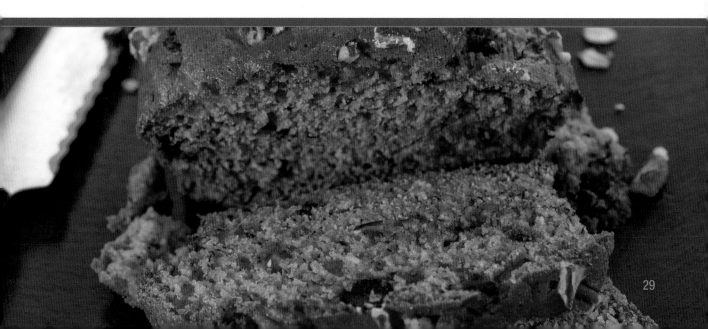

Mini BLUEBERRY PANCAKES

These charming little pancakes will get your engines roaring and fuel you for the day. Serve them with warm maple syrup.

2 cups **whole wheat flour**

1 teaspoon **baking powder**

⅛ teaspoon **salt**

2 cups unsweetened plain **soy** or **almond milk**

3 tablespoons **maple syrup**

1 tablespoon **apple cider vinegar**

1 cup fresh **blueberries**

1. Put the flour, baking powder, and salt in a large bowl and stir until well combined.

2. Add the milk, maple syrup, and vinegar and stir until smooth.

3. Warm a large nonstick skillet over medium heat for 3 minutes.

4. Lightly mist the skillet with canola oil spray.

5. Using 2 tablespoons of batter for each pancake, cook 3 to 4 pancakes at a time (depending on the size of your skillet), keeping them 1 to 2 inches apart. Arrange 5 blueberries on the top of each pancake.

6. Cook until the pancakes are golden brown on the bottom, about 4 minutes.

7. Carefully flip the pancakes over and cook the other side until golden brown, about 3 minutes.

Stored in an airtight container in the refrigerator, leftover batter will keep for about 3 days.

BUCKWHEAT Pancakes

Despite its name, buckwheat is a type of grass and is unrelated to wheat. Top these wholesome pancakes with warm maple syrup and chopped fresh fruits or whole berries.

¾ cup **buckwheat flour**

¾ cup **whole wheat pastry flour**

1 teaspoon **baking powder**

⅛ teaspoon **salt**

1¼ cups unsweetened plain **soy** or **almond milk**

¼ cup unsweetened **applesauce**

1 tablespoon **apple cider vinegar**

1 tablespoon **maple syrup**

2 teaspoons **vanilla extract**

1. Put the buckwheat flour, pastry flour, baking powder, and salt in a large bowl and stir until well combined.

2. Add the milk, applesauce, vinegar, maple syrup, and vanilla extract and stir until smooth.

3. Warm a medium nonstick skillet over medium heat for 3 minutes.

4. Lightly mist the skillet with canola oil spray.

5. Using ¼ cup of batter for each pancake, cook 2 or 3 pancakes at a time until the bottom of each pancake is golden brown, about 4 minutes.

6. Carefully flip the pancakes over and cook the other side until golden brown, about 3 minutes.

Stored in an airtight container in the refrigerator, the batter will keep for about 3 days.

WHOLE-GRAIN Waffles

f the batter is prepared in advance, these regal waffles can be on the table in ten minutes. Crown them with warm maple syrup and berries or sliced fresh fruit.

¼ cup **walnuts,** soaked in water for 4 to 5 hours and drained (see tip)

2¼ cups **water**

2 cups **rolled oats**

¼ cup **whole wheat pastry flour**

½ ripe **banana**

½ teaspoon **baking powder**

½ teaspoon **ground cinnamon**

½ teaspoon **vanilla extract**

1. Preheat an electric or standard waffle iron according to the manufacturer's instructions.

2. Put the walnuts and water in a blender and process on high speed until smooth.

3. Add the oats, flour, banana, baking powder, cinnamon, and vanilla extract and process until smooth.

4. For an electric waffle iron, cook the waffles according to the manufacturer's instructions until golden brown and crisp. For a standard waffle iron, pour a generous ½ cup of batter into the center, spreading it to within one-half inch of the edges, and close the iron. The waffle will cook in 2 to 3 minutes.

If you use a high-speed blender to process the batter, the walnuts don't need to be soaked. Stored in an airtight container in the refrigerator, the batter will keep for about 4 days.

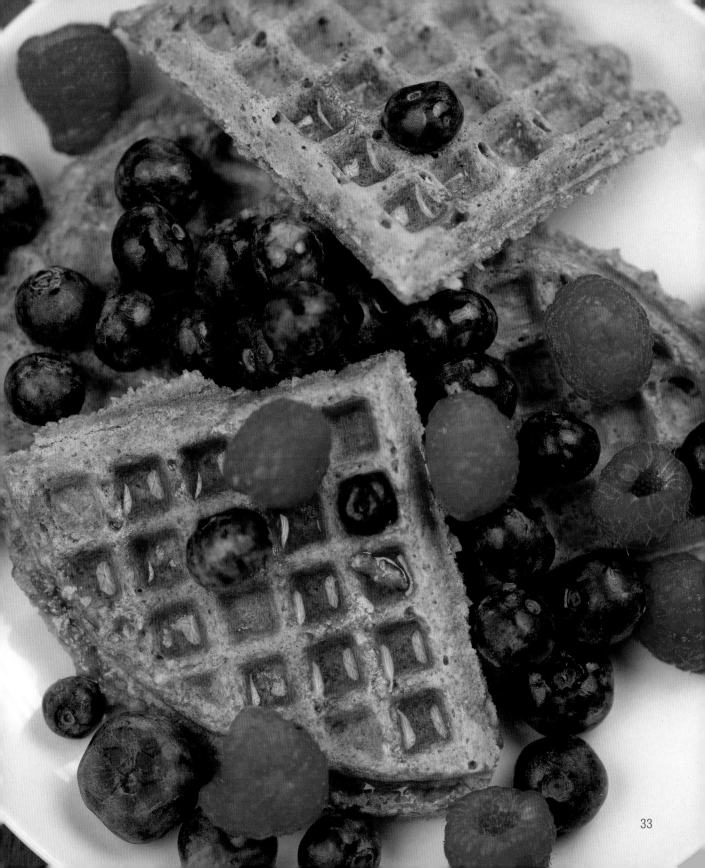

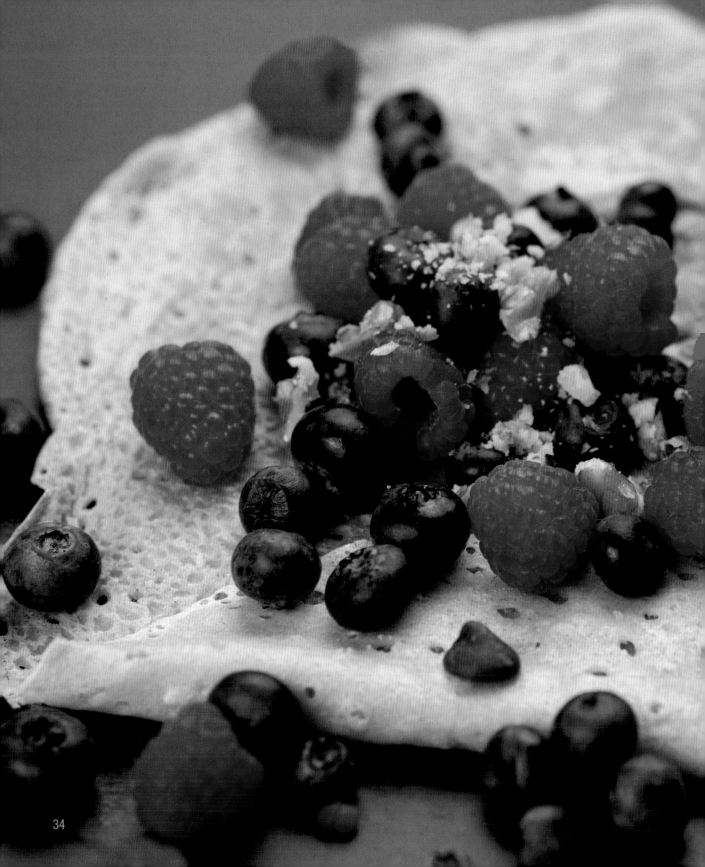

Chocolate Chip CRÊPES

No one will skip breakfast when these enchanting crêpes are on the menu. Although crêpes sound fancy, they really are a snap to prepare. For the finishing touch, embellish them with additional berries or other chopped or sliced fresh fruits, such as mangoes or peaches.

4½ cups unsweetened **soy or almond milk**

3 cups **whole wheat pastry flour**

1 teaspoon **baking powder**

1 teaspoon **vanilla extract**

¼ cup **vegan chocolate chips**

2 cups **fresh fruits** (such as blackberries, blueberries, raspberries, or sliced bananas or strawberries)

1. Put the milk, flour, baking powder, and vanilla extract in a large bowl. Beat with an electric hand mixer until smooth and well combined.

2. Warm a crêpe pan or skillet over medium heat for 3 minutes.

3. Lightly mist the pan with canola oil spray.

4. Pour ¼ cup of the batter into the pan and spread it out evenly.

5. Cook for 3 minutes, then carefully flip the crêpe over.

6. Arrange 7 or 8 chocolate chips in a line down the middle of the crêpe. The chips will partially melt while the crêpe cooks.

7. Cook for 2 minutes longer. Remove the pan from the heat and transfer the crêpe to a plate.

8. Arrange a portion of the fruit over the chocolate chips in a line down the middle of the crêpe. Roll the crêpe around the fruit and serve at once.

TIP

Stored in an airtight container in the refrigerator, the crêpe batter will keep for about 4 days.

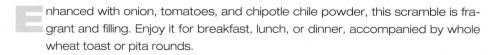

Scrambled TOFU

Enhanced with onion, tomatoes, and chipotle chile powder, this scramble is fragrant and filling. Enjoy it for breakfast, lunch, or dinner, accompanied by whole wheat toast or pita rounds.

1 (14-ounce) package **firm tofu**

½ cup finely chopped **red onion**

1½ **Roma tomatoes,** finely chopped

½ teaspoon **salt**

¼ teaspoon **chipotle chile powder**

¼ cup finely chopped **fresh cilantro,** lightly packed

1 Put the tofu in a medium bowl and crumble it using your hands or the back of a fork. Set aside.

2 Warm a medium skillet over medium-high heat for 3 minutes.

3 Lightly mist the skillet with canola oil spray.

4 Put the onion in the hot skillet and cook, stirring frequently, until lightly browned, about 4 minutes.

5 Add the tomatoes, salt, and chile powder and stir to combine. Cover and cook until the tomatoes soften, about 8 minutes.

6 Stir the tofu into the tomato mixture and cook, stirring occasionally, until the tofu is hot, about 4 minutes.

7 Sprinkle with the cilantro just before serving.

Stored in an airtight container in the refrigerator, the scramble will keep for about 4 days. Reheat in the microwave or on the stove top before serving.

BULGUR Pudding

Bulgur is made from finely chopped wheat berries that are partially boiled and dried before being packaged. For this unique breakfast dish, bulgur is transformed into a soothing pudding that will keep your hunger at bay until lunchtime.

4 cups **water**

1½ cups coarse **bulgur**

⅛ teaspoon **salt**

2 cups unsweetened **soy** or **almond milk**

⅓ cup **raisins**

⅓ cup **sugar**

2 tablespoons sliced or slivered **almonds**

½ teaspoon **ground cardamom**

Stored in an airtight container in the refrigerator, the pudding will keep for about 4 days. Leftover pudding tastes best when served warm. However, the bulgur will absorb the milk over time. Add more milk as needed prior to warming the pudding on the stove top.

1. Put the water, bulgur, and salt in a medium saucepan and bring to a boil over high heat.

2. Decrease the heat to low, cover, and cook until the bulgur is soft, about 15 minutes. Remove from the heat.

3. Add the milk, raisins, sugar, almonds, and cardamom and stir until evenly combined. Serve warm.

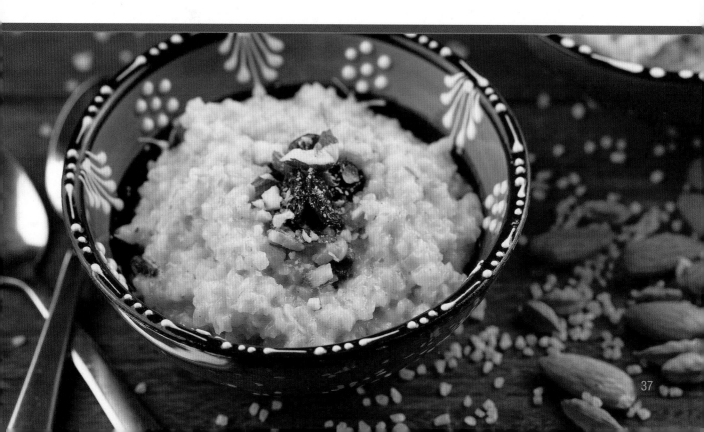

5
Salads

Hearty Salad

Tomato and Cucumber SALAD

MAKES 4 SERVINGS

This simple salad is a first-rate complement to rich-tasting dishes, such as Curried Black-Eyed Peas (page 64) and Aloo Gobi (page 119).

1 cup finely chopped **tomato**

1 cup finely chopped **cucumber**

½ cup finely chopped **white onion**

½ teaspoon freshly squeezed **lemon** or **lime juice**

⅛ teaspoon **salt**

Ground **black pepper**

1. Put the tomato, cucumber, onion, lemon juice, and salt in a medium bowl and stir until well combined.

2. Season with pepper to taste.

Stored in an airtight container in the refrigerator, the salad will keep for about 3 days.

BRUSCHETTA

MAKES 4 SERVINGS

Bruschetta is a sweet-and-tangy Italian appetizer made with fresh tomatoes, fresh basil, and balsamic vinegar. Spread it generously over toasted slices of whole-grain bread.

1½ pints (3 cups) **grape tomatoes,** sliced in half

3 small **garlic cloves,** peeled and crushed

2 tablespoons **balsamic vinegar**

6 large **basil leaves,** finely chopped

¼ teaspoon **salt**

1. Put all the ingredients in a large bowl and stir until well combined.

2. Refrigerate for at least 1 hour before serving to allow the flavors to blend.

Stored in an airtight container in the refrigerator, the bruschetta will keep for 2 to 3 days. Serve at room temperature.

Pasta SALAD

Whole-grain pasta, legumes, vegetables, and fresh fruits form the basis of this unique salad, which is simultaneously savory, tangy, and slightly sweet.

4 ounces **whole wheat fusilli**

¾ cup halved seedless **grapes**

¾ cup unsalted cooked or canned **chickpeas,** rinsed and drained

½ cup finely chopped **cucumber**

¼ cup finely chopped **celery**

8 pitted **kalamata olives**

1 tablespoon finely chopped **white onion**

Salt

Ground **black pepper**

Freshly squeezed **lemon** or **lime juice**

1 Cook the fusilli according to the package directions. Rinse with cold water to cool it quickly. Drain well.

2 Put the fusilli, grapes, chickpeas, cucumber, celery, olives, and onion in a large bowl and gently toss to combine.

3 Season with salt, pepper, and lemon juice to taste and gently toss until evenly distributed.

Stored in an airtight container in the refrigerator, the salad will keep for about 3 days. Serve at room temperature.

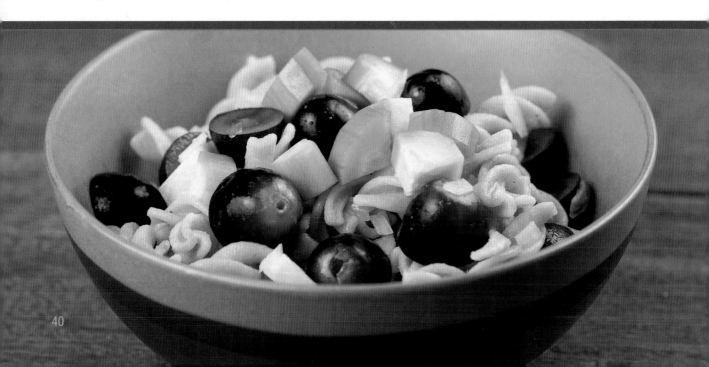

40

Couscous SALAD

Light but satisfying, this salad is best enjoyed at room temperature, making it an excellent choice for school or work lunches, picnics, or travel days.

1 cup **whole wheat couscous**

1 cup finely chopped **tomato**

¾ cup unsalted cooked or canned **chickpeas,** rinsed and drained

½ cup finely chopped **cucumber**

¼ cup finely chopped **white onion**

8 pitted **kalamata olives**

Salt

Ground **black pepper**

Freshly squeezed **lemon** or **lime juice**

1. Cook the couscous according to the package instructions.

2. Put the cooked couscous, tomato, chickpeas, cucumber, onion, and olives in a large bowl and gently stir to combine.

3. Season with salt, pepper, and lemon juice to taste.

Stored in an airtight container in the refrigerator, the salad will keep for about 3 days. Serve at room temperature.

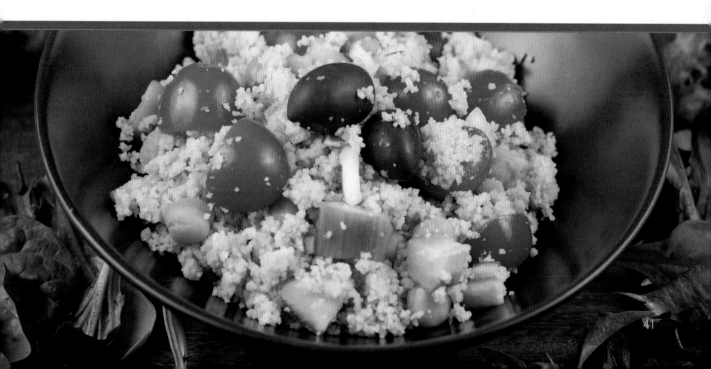

HEARTY Salad

Chickpeas and pasta team up to create a substantial salad that can stand on its own as a meal.

4 ounces **whole wheat fusilli**

1 (15-ounce) can unsalted **chickpeas,** rinsed and drained

1 (5-ounce) package **salad greens**

12 pitted **kalamata olives**

½ cup diced **cucumber**

½ cup halved or quartered **grape** or **cherry tomatoes**

¼ cup thinly sliced **onion**

½ cup **Hummus Dressing** (page 82) or **Low-Fat Creamy Salad Dressing** (page 80)

Stored in an airtight container in the refrigerator, the salad will keep for about 2 days.

1 Cook the fusilli according to the package directions. Rinse with cold water to cool it quickly. Drain well.

2 Put the fusilli, chickpeas, salad greens, olives, cucumber, tomatoes, and onion in a large salad bowl and gently toss until well combined.

3 Add the dressing and toss until evenly distributed.

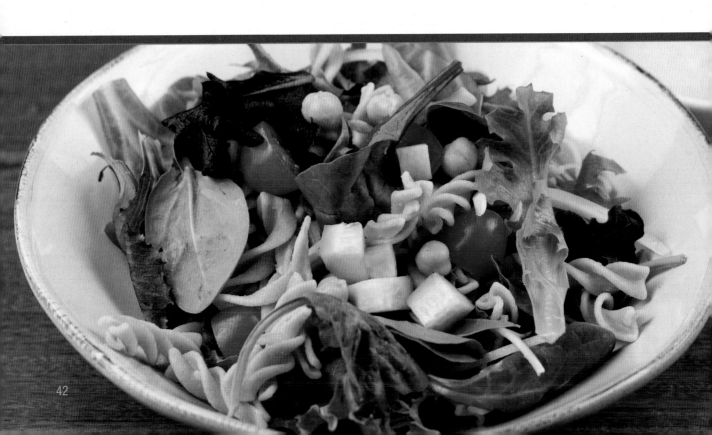

Mediterranean CHICKPEA SALAD

Refreshing and filling, this salad makes an excellent side dish for lighter fare and is a good choice when hunger strikes midday.

8 cups unsalted cooked or canned **chickpeas,** rinsed and drained

½ cup finely chopped **scallions**

¼ cup finely chopped **fresh parsley,** lightly packed

3 tablespoons **white wine vinegar**

1 tablespoon finely chopped **fresh dill**

1 tablespoon **olive oil**

1 teaspoon **salt**

1 Put all the ingredients in a large bowl and stir until well combined.

2 Refrigerate for at least 1 hour before serving to allow the flavors to blend.

Stored in an airtight container in the refrigerator, the salad will keep for about 4 days. Serve at room temperature.

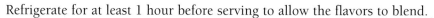

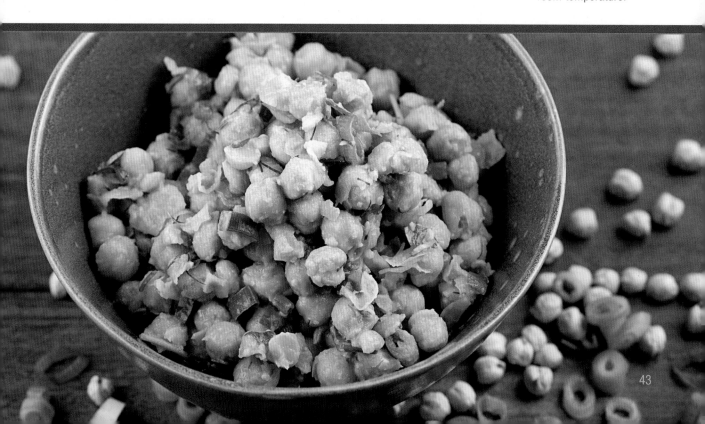

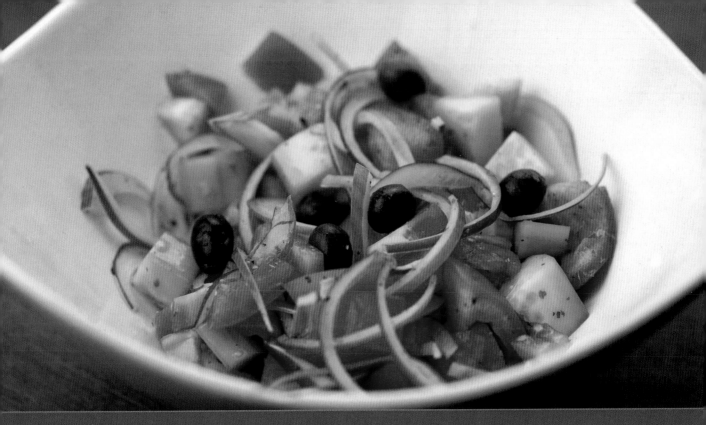

Greek Salad *(above)*

(below) **Salsa Fresca**

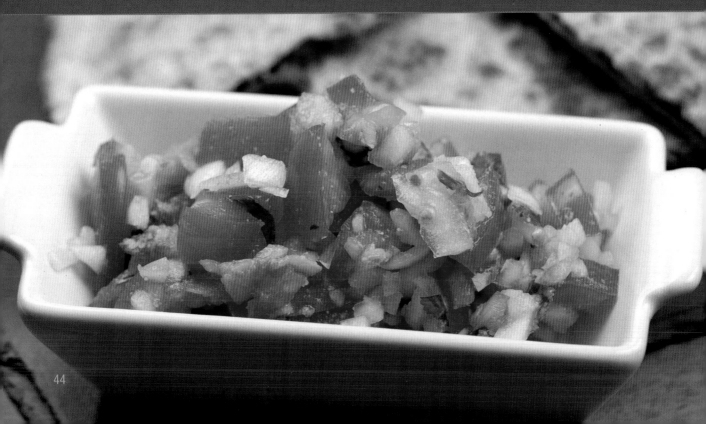

Greek SALAD

MAKES 4 SERVINGS

This simple salad has a surprising depth and partners well with virtually any entrée.

2 **tomatoes,** diced

½ medium **cucumber,** peeled and diced

12 pitted **kalamata olives**

⅛ medium **red onion,** thinly sliced

1½ tablespoons **red wine vinegar**

½ teaspoon **salt**

½ teaspoon **dried oregano**

1 Put all the ingredients in a large salad bowl and gently stir until well combined.

2 Serve chilled or at room temperature.

Stored in an airtight container in the refrigerator, the salad will keep for about 3 days.

SALSA Fresca

MAKES 4 CUPS, 6 SERVINGS

This cooling, no-cook relish augments a wide range of Mexican-style dishes.

6 **Roma tomatoes,** finely chopped

¼ cup finely chopped **white onion**

¼ cup finely chopped **fresh cilantro**

2 teaspoons freshly squeezed **lemon** or **lime juice**

¾ teaspoon **garlic granules**

½ teaspoon **salt**

Finely chopped **jalapeño chiles,** for garnish

1 Put the tomatoes, onion, cilantro, lemon juice, garlic granules, and salt in a large bowl and stir until well combined.

2 Garnish with jalapeño chiles just before serving.

Stored in an airtight container in the refrigerator, the salsa will keep for about 3 days.

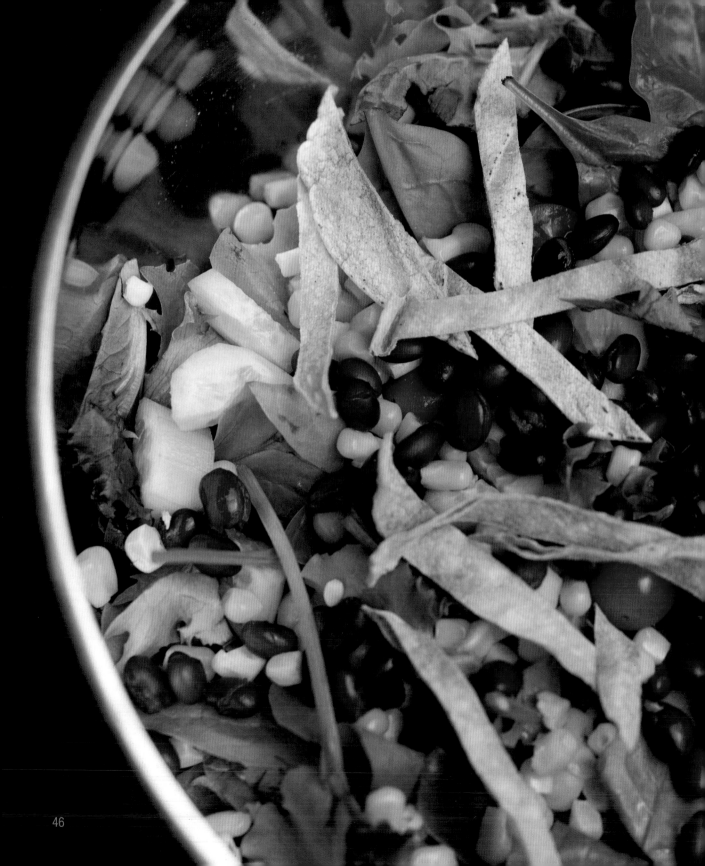

Tex-Mex Salad WITH BLACK BEANS

To compose this captivating salad, toss together black beans, veggies, and a delectable dressing, then top with crunchy baked tortilla crisps just before serving.

4 **corn tortillas**

1 cup frozen **corn kernels**

2½ cups **water**

1 (15-ounce) can unsalted **black beans,** rinsed and drained

1 (5-ounce) package **salad greens**

½ cup halved or quartered **grape** or **cherry tomatoes**

½ cup diced **cucumber**

¼ cup thinly sliced **onion**

½ cup **Peanut-Cilantro Salad Dressing** (page 81), plus more as needed

1. Preheat the oven to 400 degrees F. Line a baking sheet with parchment paper.

2. Slice the tortillas into ½-inch-wide strips.

3. Arrange the tortilla strips in a single layer on the lined baking sheet and bake for 7 to 8 minutes, until lightly browned. Adjust the baking time as needed, depending on your oven and the thickness of the tortillas.

4. Remove the tortilla strips from the oven and let cool on a rack. They will become crispier as they cool.

5. Put the corn and water in a small saucepan and bring to a boil over high heat. Decrease the heat to medium-high and cook until the corn is soft, about 5 minutes. Drain in a colander in the sink. Rinse with cold water and drain again.

6. Put the corn, beans, salad greens, tomatoes, cucumber, and onion in a large salad bowl and gently toss to combine. Add the dressing and gently toss until evenly distributed. Add more dressing to taste, if desired.

7. Top with the crispy tortilla strips just before serving.

Stored in separate airtight containers, the salad will keep in the refrigerator for about 2 days and the tortilla crisps will keep at room temperature for about 2 days.

Green Pea and Avocado Dip

GREEN PEA AND AVOCADO Dip

MAKES 3 CUPS, 6 SERVINGS

The sweetness of peas and the creaminess of avocado converge in this low-fat, decadent-tasting dip. Dive in with baked tortilla chips, toasted whole wheat pita bread, or toast points.

16 ounces (1 pound) frozen **peas**

Pulp of 1 ripe **avocado**

2 tablespoons freshly squeezed **lemon** or **lime juice**

1 tablespoon **garlic granules**

¾ teaspoon **salt**

¼ cup finely chopped **white onion**

1 Put the peas in a medium saucepan and cover with water. Bring to a boil over high heat (do not cover). Decrease the heat to medium-high and cook uncovered until the peas are soft, about 5 minutes. Drain the peas in a colander in the sink, rinse with cold water, and drain again.

2 Put the peas, avocado pulp, lemon juice, garlic granules, and salt in a blender and pulse until slightly chunky.

3 Spoon into a large bowl and stir in the onion.

Stored in an airtight container in the refrigerator, the dip will keep for about 2 days.

CLASSIC Guacamole

MAKES 2 CUPS, 6 SERVINGS

This luxurious guacamole makes a splendid accompaniment to spicy south-of-the-border dishes, such as Black Bean Tacos (page 124), Nacho Platter (page 126), Burrito Bowls (page 127), and Mexican Casserole (page 128).

Pulp of 2 ripe **avocados**

¼ cup finely chopped **onion**

1 tablespoon finely chopped **fresh cilantro**

¼ teaspoon **garlic granules**

2 teaspoons freshly squeezed **lemon** or **lime juice**

¼ teaspoon **salt**

Finely chopped **jalapeño chiles**, for garnish

1 Put the avocado pulp in a large bowl and mash with a fork until slightly chunky.

2 Add the onion, cilantro, lemon juice, garlic granules, and salt and stir with a fork until well combined.

3 Garnish with jalapeño chiles just before serving.

Guacamole is best served fresh. Stored in an airtight container in the refrigerator, the guacamole will keep for 24 to 48 hours. Scrape off the top brown layer before serving.

ROASTED GARLIC Hummus

This nutritious Middle Eastern dip can be enjoyed with crackers or raw veggies or used as a sandwich spread. Roasted garlic kicks the flavor into high gear, minimizing the need for added fat.

2 **garlic cloves,** peeled

1 can unsalted **chickpeas,** rinsed and drained

¼ cup **water,** plus more as needed

3 tablespoons **tahini**

1½ tablespoons freshly squeezed **lemon** or **lime juice**

½ teaspoon **salt**

1 Warm a small nonstick pan over medium heat for 3 minutes.

2 Lightly mist the surface of the pan with canola oil spray and roast the garlic in the pan until golden brown, about 3 minutes. Turn the garlic every 1 to 2 minutes to ensure even roasting.

3 Put the garlic, chickpeas, water, tahini, lemon juice, and salt in a blender and process until smooth. Add a little more water if the hummus is too thick.

Stored in an airtight container in the refrigerator, the hummus will keep for about 4 days.

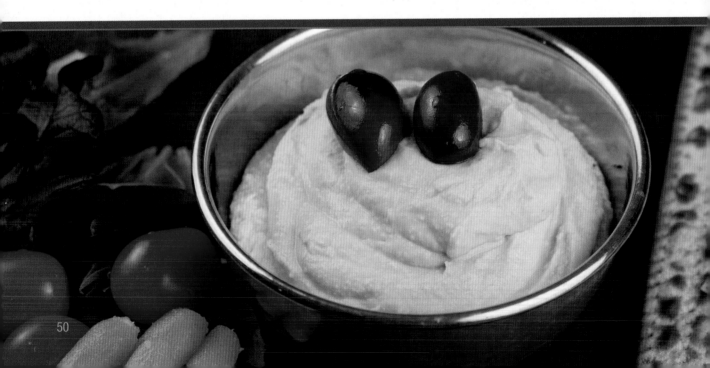

Edamame **HUMMUS**

MAKES 2½ CUPS, 6 SERVINGS

This rich, creamy hummus is packed with protein. Serve it with toasted whole wheat pita triangles for dipping or use it as a spread for veggie sandwiches.

2 cups frozen shelled **edamame**

2 **garlic cloves,** peeled

½ cup **water,** plus more as needed

2 tablespoons **tahini**

1½ tablespoons freshly squeezed **lemon** or **lime juice**

½ teaspoon **salt**

1. Put the edamame in a medium saucepan and cover with water. Bring to a boil over high heat (do not cover). Decrease the heat to medium-high and cook uncovered until the edamame is soft, about 9 minutes. Drain the edamame in a colander in the sink, rinse with cold water, and drain again.

2. Warm a small nonstick pan over medium heat for 3 minutes.

3. Lightly mist the surface of the pan with canola oil spray and roast the garlic in the pan until golden brown, about 3 minutes. Turn the garlic every 1 to 2 minutes to ensure even roasting.

4. Put the edamame, garlic, water, tahini, lemon juice, and salt in a blender and process until smooth. Add a little more water if the hummus is too thick.

Stored in an airtight container in the refrigerator, the hummus will keep for about 4 days.

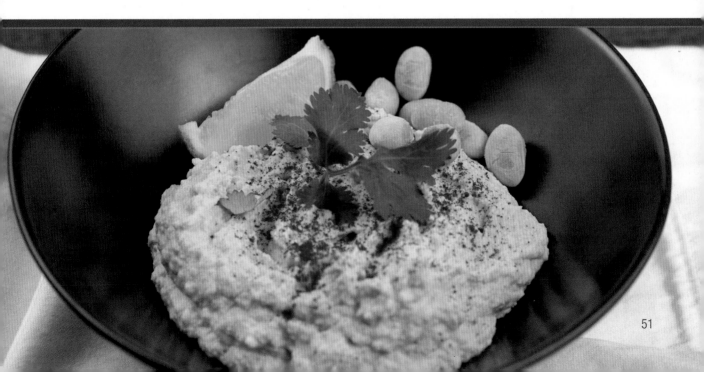

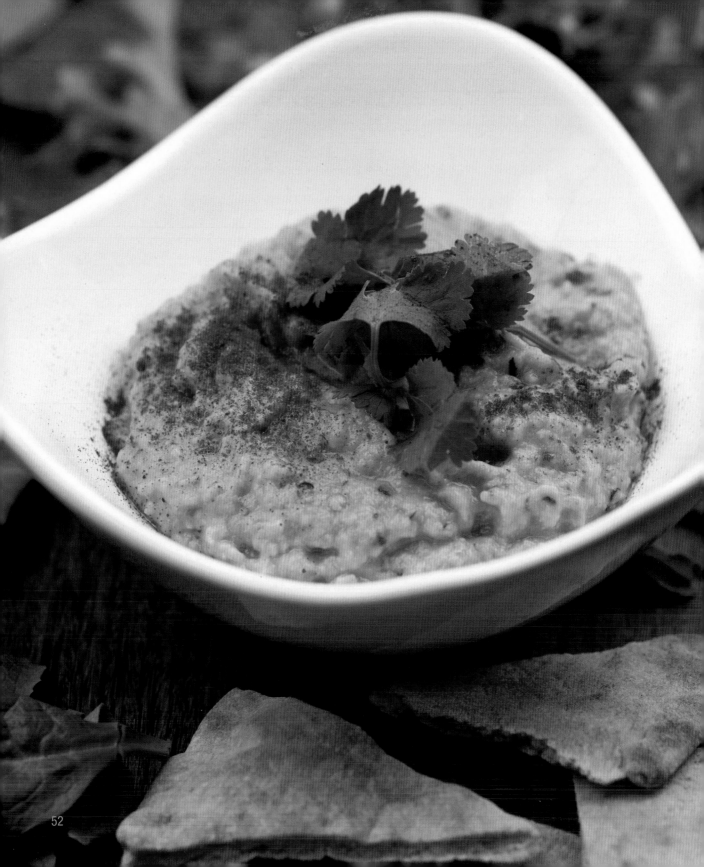

Baba Ghanoush (ROASTED EGGPLANT DIP)

MAKES 2 CUPS, 6 SERVINGS

For a superb appetizer or snack, serve this famous Middle Eastern staple with whole wheat pita bread or toasted whole wheat pita chips.

1 large purple **eggplant**

5 **garlic cloves,** peeled

1½ tablespoons **tahini**

½ teaspoon **salt,** plus more as needed

¼ teaspoon **sumac,** for garnish (see tip)

1 tablespoon finely chopped **fresh parsley,** for garnish

1. Preheat the oven to 425 degrees F.

2. Wash the eggplant, pat it dry, and lay it down in a baking dish. Make a small cut on the top side of the eggplant with a knife so that it doesn't burst while baking.

3. Bake the eggplant for 1 hour, until the skin is crisp and the interior is soft.

4. Remove the eggplant from the oven and let cool on a rack for about 30 minutes.

5. After the eggplant has cooled, slice it open. Scoop out the pulp with a spoon and put it in a blender, leaving the skin behind.

6. Warm a small nonstick pan over medium heat for 3 minutes.

7. Lightly mist the surface of the pan with canola oil spray and roast the garlic in the pan until brown, about 5 minutes. Turn the garlic every 1 to 2 minutes to ensure even roasting.

8. Add the garlic, tahini, and salt to the eggplant in the blender and pulse until the dip is slightly chunky. Taste and add more salt if needed.

9. Garnish with the sumac and parsley just before serving.

Sumac is a Mediterranean spice prized for its sharp, citrusy flavor. If you are unable to find it locally, look for it online. Stored in an airtight container in the refrigerator, the dip will keep for about 4 days.

Broccoli and Chickpea-Cheddar DIP

MAKES 8 CUPS, 6 SERVINGS

This brightly colored, high-protein mashup makes an uplifting snack or even a light meal when served with toasted whole wheat bread or pita rounds.

2 (15-ounce) cans unsalted **chickpeas,** rinsed and drained

2½ cups unsweetened plain **soy** or **almond milk**

⅓ cup **nutritional yeast flakes**

½ cup **almond flour**

2 tablespoons freshly squeezed **lemon** or **lime juice**

2 tablespoons **tapioca starch**

2 teaspoons **garlic granules**

2 teaspoons **onion powder**

1½ teaspoons **salt**

1 teaspoon **smoked paprika**

1 teaspoon crushed **red chile flakes**

6 cups finely chopped **broccoli**

1. Preheat the oven to 375 degrees F. Line a 10-inch round cake pan with parchment paper.

2. Put the chickpeas, milk, nutritional yeast, almond flour, lemon juice, tapioca starch, garlic granules, onion powder, salt, paprika, and chile flakes in a blender and process until smooth.

3. Put the broccoli in the lined pan and cover with the blended mixture. Gently stir to combine.

4. Bake uncovered for 25 minutes, until the top is golden brown.

Stored in an airtight container in the refrigerator, the dip will keep for about 4 days. Just before serving, reheat until warm in the microwave or in the oven at 350 degrees F.

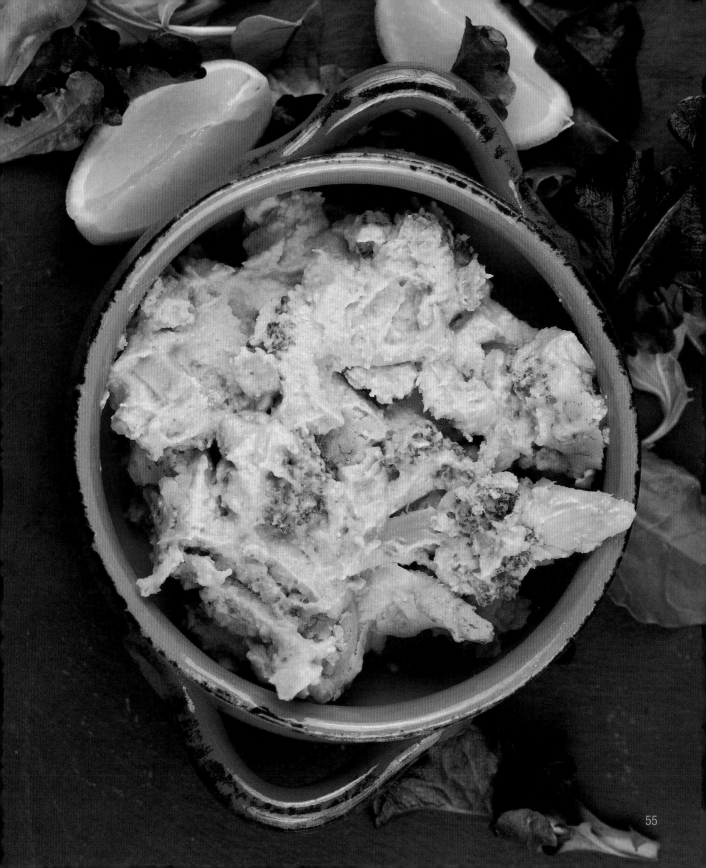

Muhammara 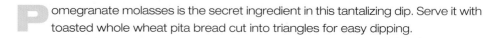 (ROASTED RED PEPPER DIP)

MAKES 2½ CUPS, 6 SERVINGS

Pomegranate molasses is the secret ingredient in this tantalizing dip. Serve it with toasted whole wheat pita bread cut into triangles for easy dipping.

3 large **red bell peppers**

2 slices **whole wheat bread,** toasted and torn into pieces

½ cup crumbled **extra-firm tofu,** or ¼ cup **walnuts**

1 tablespoon **pomegranate molasses**

1 **garlic clove,** peeled and crushed

½ teaspoon **ground cumin**

½ teaspoon **salt**

1 Preheat the oven to 350 degrees F. Line a medium baking pan with parchment paper.

2 Put the whole peppers in the lined baking pan and roast in the oven for 35 minutes. Turn the peppers occasionally to ensure even roasting. Let cool for 15 minutes, then remove the stems and seeds.

3 Put the peppers, bread, tofu, pomegranate molasses, garlic, cumin, and salt in a blender and pulse until slightly chunky.

Stored in an airtight container in the refrigerator, the dip will keep for about 4 days.

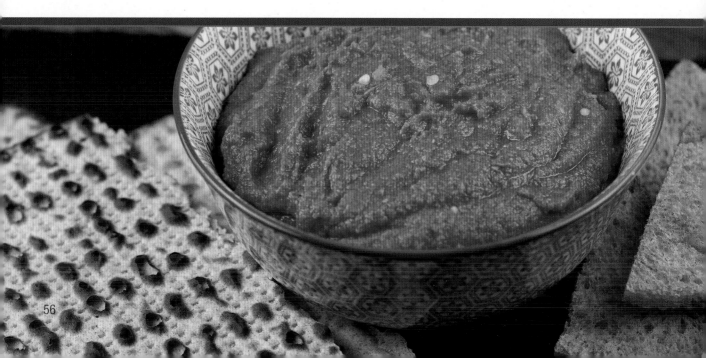

Creamy SPINACH-ARTICHOKE DIP

MAKES 6 CUPS, 8 SERVINGS

Chickpeas, artichokes, spinach, and seasonings meld beautifully to produce a healthier version of this exalted dip. It makes a gratifying snack or light meal when teamed with whole-grain toast points or baked tortilla chips.

1 (15-ounce) can unsalted **chickpeas,** rinsed and drained

1¼ cups unsweetened plain **soy** or **almond milk**

⅓ cup raw **cashews**

¼ cup **nutritional yeast flakes**

3 tablespoons freshly squeezed **lemon** or **lime juice**

1 tablespoon **garlic granules**

1¼ teaspoons **salt**

¾ teaspoon crushed **red chile flakes**

¾ (12-ounce) package frozen **artichoke hearts** (see tip)

½ (5-ounce) package fresh **baby spinach**

1 Preheat the oven to 400 degrees F. Line an 8-inch square baking pan with parchment paper.

2 Put the chickpeas, milk, cashews, nutritional yeast, lemon juice, garlic granules, salt, and chile flakes in a high-speed blender or food processor and process until smooth.

3 Gradually add the artichokes and spinach and pulse to create a chunky texture.

4 Pour into the lined baking pan and bake for 35 minutes, until the top is golden brown.

Let the artichoke hearts sit at room temperature for 20 minutes prior to using so they can defrost. Stored in an airtight container in the refrigerator, the dip will keep for about 4 days. Just before serving, reheat until warm in the microwave or in the oven at 350 degrees F.

*Italian Brown Lentil Soup
with Vegetables*

GAZPACHO

Gazpacho is an invigorating Spanish-style soup that is traditionally served well chilled. The crispy croutons in this recipe elevate it to the next level.

2 pounds **tomatoes** or **Roma tomatoes**

8 ounces **cucumbers,** peeled

¼ **white onion,** peeled

¼ cup **water,** plus more as needed

3 tablespoons **red wine vinegar,** plus more as needed

1 tablespoon **olive oil**

1 teaspoon **salt,** plus more as needed

1 **garlic clove,** peeled

5 slices **whole wheat bread,** cut into ½-inch cubes

1 To make the gazpacho, put the tomatoes, cucumbers, onion, water, vinegar, oil, salt, and garlic in a high-speed blender or food processor and process until slightly chunky. Add a little more water if the soup is very thick. Add more salt and vinegar to taste.

2 Chill in the refrigerator for at least 12 hours before serving to allow the flavors to blend.

3 To make the croutons, preheat the oven to 400 degrees F.

4 Spread the bread cubes in a single layer on a baking sheet and bake for 10 minutes, until golden brown. Let cool.

5 Top the soup with the croutons just before serving.

Stored in an airtight container in the refrigerator, the soup will keep for 3 to 4 days. Stored at room temperature in an airtight container, the croutons will keep for about 3 days.

Veggie CHILI

This robust chili comes together within minutes. To round out your meal, ladle it over baked potatoes, whole wheat pasta, or baked tortilla chips.

3 cups **Restaurant-Style Salsa** (page 79)

2½ cups cooked or canned unsalted **black beans,** rinsed and drained

1½ cups frozen **corn kernels**

Stored in an airtight container in the refrigerator, the chili will keep for about 4 days.

1 Put all the ingredients in a medium saucepan and stir until well combined.

2 Bring to a boil over medium-high heat. Decrease the heat to medium and simmer, stirring occasionally, for 10 minutes.

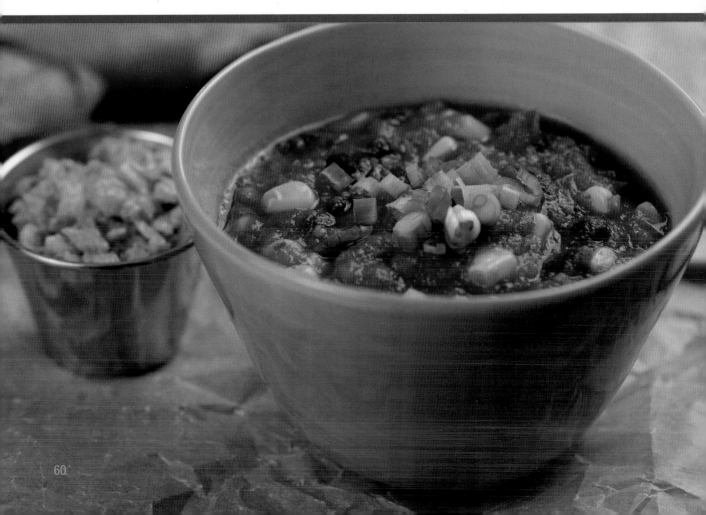

Chana Masala (CHICKPEA STEW)

Chickpeas are combined with a judicious blend of herbs and spices in this richly seasoned North Indian stew. Mashed chickpeas thicken the sauce and impart a creamy consistency without any added fat. Serve it with brown rice, bulgur, or quinoa on the side.

3 cups finely chopped **onions**

3 cups finely chopped **tomatoes**

2 tablespoons crushed **garlic**

½ teaspoon grated **fresh ginger**

2 teaspoons **cumin seeds**

1½ teaspoons **salt**

1 teaspoon **cayenne**

1 teaspoon **ground coriander**

½ teaspoon **ground turmeric**

½ teaspoon **garam masala**

6 cups unsalted cooked or canned **chickpeas,** rinsed and drained

4 cups **water,** plus more as needed

Lemon wedges, for garnish

Finely chopped **green chiles,** for garnish

Finely chopped **fresh cilantro,** for garnish

1. Warm a large saucepan over medium-high heat for 3 minutes.

2. Lightly mist the skillet with canola oil spray.

3. Put the onions in the skillet and cook, stirring frequently, until golden brown, about 4 minutes.

4. Add the tomatoes, garlic, and ginger and cook, stirring frequently, for 4 minutes.

5. Add the cumin seeds, salt, cayenne, coriander, turmeric, and garam masala and stir until well combined. Cover and cook, stirring frequently, until the tomatoes are very soft, about 7 minutes.

6. Add the chickpeas and water and stir to combine. Bring to a boil. Decrease the heat to medium and cook, stirring occasionally, until the chickpeas are very soft, about 8 minutes.

7. Use a potato masher or the back of a sturdy slotted spoon to mash some of the chickpeas against the bottom or side of the pan.

8. If the stew is very thick, add water in ½-cup increments until it has thinned slightly. If the stew is watery, increase the heat and simmer until it has thickened slightly. Remove from the heat.

9. Garnish with lemon wedges, chiles, and cilantro just before serving.

Stored in an airtight container, the stew will keep in the refrigerator for about 4 days or in the freezer for about 6 weeks.

MINESTRONE

Brimming with veggies, legumes, and whole grains, this soup is a nutritional rock star. Subtle seasonings unite the ingredients to create an impressive rendition of this beloved Italian specialty.

8 ounces **whole wheat elbow macaroni** or **fusilli**

1 unpeeled **potato,** finely chopped

1 teaspoon **olive oil**

1 **red onion,** finely chopped

10 **garlic cloves,** peeled and crushed

2 cups shredded or finely chopped **carrots**

2 **zucchini,** finely chopped, or 3 cups finely chopped **kale,** firmly packed

2 teaspoons **salt**

1 (15-ounce) can unsalted **chickpeas,** rinsed and drained

1½ cups frozen **corn kernels**

¼ cup plus 3 tablespoons unsalted **tomato paste**

5 cups **water**

2 teaspoons **Italian seasoning**

1 Cook the pasta according to the package directions and set aside.

2 Put the potatoes and ½ cup of water in a microwave-safe bowl and microwave until the potatoes are soft, about 3 minutes. Alternatively, put the potatoes and ½ cup of water in a small saucepan and simmer on the stove top over medium-high heat until soft, about 10 minutes. Remove from the heat and drain. Set aside.

3 Put the oil in a large saucepan over medium-high heat until warm, 2 to 3 minutes.

4 Add the onion and garlic and cook, stirring frequently, until golden brown, 3 to 4 minutes.

5 Add the carrots, zucchini (if using), and salt. Cover and cook, stirring frequently, until the carrots are soft, about 5 minutes.

6 Add the chickpeas, kale (if using), corn, and tomato paste and stir until well combined. Cover and cook, stirring frequently, for 3 minutes.

7 Add the water and bring to a boil. Boil for 2 minutes. Remove from the heat and stir in the Italian seasoning.

8 Top with the pasta just before serving.

Store the pasta and soup in separate containers to prevent the pasta from absorbing the liquid from the soup. Stored in airtight containers in the refrigerator, the soup and pasta will each keep for 3 to 4 days.

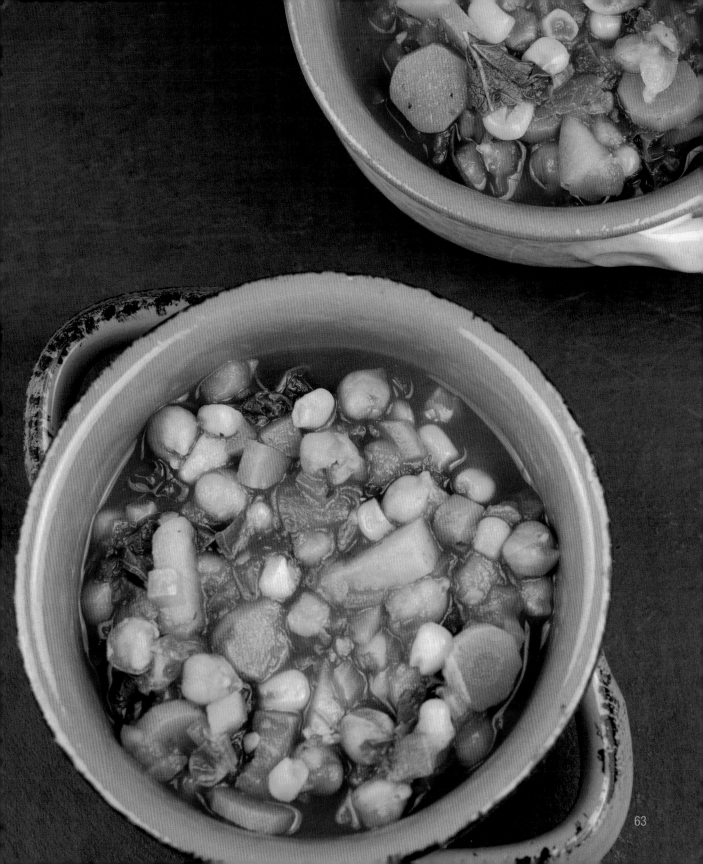

Curried BLACK-EYED PEAS

Black-eyed peas are rich in protein and fiber. Serve this exquisite curry over brown rice or bulgur.

1 cup finely chopped **onion**

2 cups finely chopped **tomatoes**

2 teaspoons **cumin seeds**

1 teaspoon **cayenne**

1 teaspoon **ground coriander**

1 teaspoon **salt**

½ teaspoon **ground turmeric**

½ teaspoon **garam masala**

4 cups cooked or canned unsalted **black-eyed peas**, rinsed and drained

4 cups **water**, plus more as needed

Lemon wedges, for garnish

Finely chopped **green chiles**, for garnish

Finely chopped **fresh cilantro**, for garnish

1. Warm a large saucepan over medium-high heat for 3 minutes.

2. Lightly mist the surface of the pan with canola oil spray.

3. Put the onion in the pan and cook over medium heat, stirring occasionally, until golden brown, about 4 minutes.

4. Add the tomatoes and stir to combine. Cover and cook, stirring occasionally, for 4 minutes.

5. Add the cumin seeds, cayenne, coriander, salt, turmeric, and garam masala and stir until well combined. Cover and cook, stirring occasionally, until the tomatoes are very soft, about 7 minutes.

6. Add the black-eyed peas and water and stir to combine. Increase the heat to medium-high and bring to a boil. Decrease the heat to medium and cook, stirring occasionally, for 8 minutes.

7. If the sauce is very thick, add water in ½-cup increments until it has thinned slightly. If the sauce is watery, increase the heat and simmer until the sauce has thickened slightly.

8. Garnish with lemon wedges, green chiles, and cilantro just before serving.

Stored in an airtight container, the curry will keep in the refrigerator for about 4 days or in the freezer for about 6 weeks.

Cannellini Beans WITH VEGETABLES

Meaty cannellini beans, also known as white kidney beans or great Northern beans, are seasoned with a variety of herbs and vegetables to create an opulent stew.

2 tablespoons crushed **garlic**

2 cups finely chopped **celery**

2 cups shredded **carrots**

5 cups **water**

3 tablespoons unsalted **tomato paste**

2 teaspoons **salt**

1½ teaspoons **dried oregano**

1½ teaspoons **dried thyme**

3 (15-ounce) cans unsalted **cannellini beans,** rinsed and drained

1 tablespoon **sherry vinegar**

⅓ cup finely chopped **parsley,** lightly packed, for garnish

1 Warm a large saucepan over medium heat for 2 minutes.

2 Lightly mist the surface of the pan with canola oil spray.

3 Put the garlic in the pan and cook, stirring frequently, until golden brown, about 2 minutes.

4 Add the celery and carrots and stir until well combined. Cover and cook for 1 minute.

5 Add the water, tomato paste, salt, oregano, and thyme and stir until well combined. Cover and cook until the carrots are soft, about 8 minutes.

6 Add the beans and stir to combine.

7 Bring to a boil over medium-high heat, stirring occasionally.

8 Remove from the heat and stir in the vinegar until well incorporated.

9 Garnish with the parsley just before serving.

Stored in an airtight container in the refrigerator, the stew will keep for about 4 days.

Moorish CHICKPEA STEW

This aromatic, Spanish-inspired stew is chock-full of goodness. Complement it with toasted baguette slices on the side.

12 ounces (1½ cups) dried **chickpeas,** rinsed, drained, and soaked in water for 8 to 12 hours

1 teaspoon **olive oil**

7 **garlic cloves,** peeled and crushed

1 teaspoon **cumin seeds**

1 teaspoon **smoked Spanish paprika** or **smoked paprika**

1 teaspoon **salt**

8 ounces **baby spinach,** or 8 ounces **curly kale,** finely chopped

2 tablespoons **sherry vinegar**

1. Drain and rinse the chickpeas. Put them in a medium saucepan, add enough fresh water to cover the chickpeas completely, and bring to a boil over medium-high heat. Decrease the heat to medium and simmer until the chickpeas are tender, about 45 minutes. Remove from the heat and set aside.

2. Warm the oil in a medium saucepan over medium heat for 2 minutes.

3. Add the garlic and cumin seeds and cook, stirring frequently, until golden brown, about 3 minutes.

4. Add the paprika and salt and cook, stirring constantly, for 30 seconds.

5. Add the chickpeas and their cooking liquid and stir to combine. Cover and bring to a simmer over medium heat. Cook, stirring occasionally, for 15 minutes. Add water as needed to ensure there is enough sauce around the chickpeas.

6. Use a potato masher or the back of a sturdy slotted spoon to mash some of the chickpeas against the bottom or side of the pan.

7. If the stew is very thick, add water in ½-cup increments until it has thinned slightly. If the stew is watery, increase the heat and simmer until it has thickened slightly.

8. Remove from heat. Add the spinach and vinegar and stir until the spinach is wilted and all the ingredients are well combined.

Stored in an airtight container in the refrigerator, the stew will keep for about 4 days.

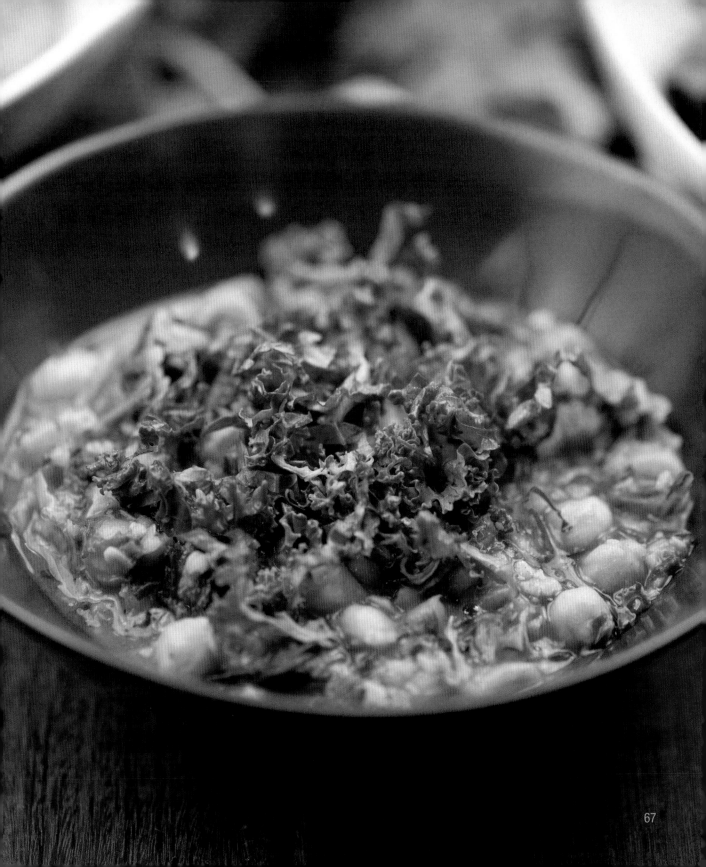

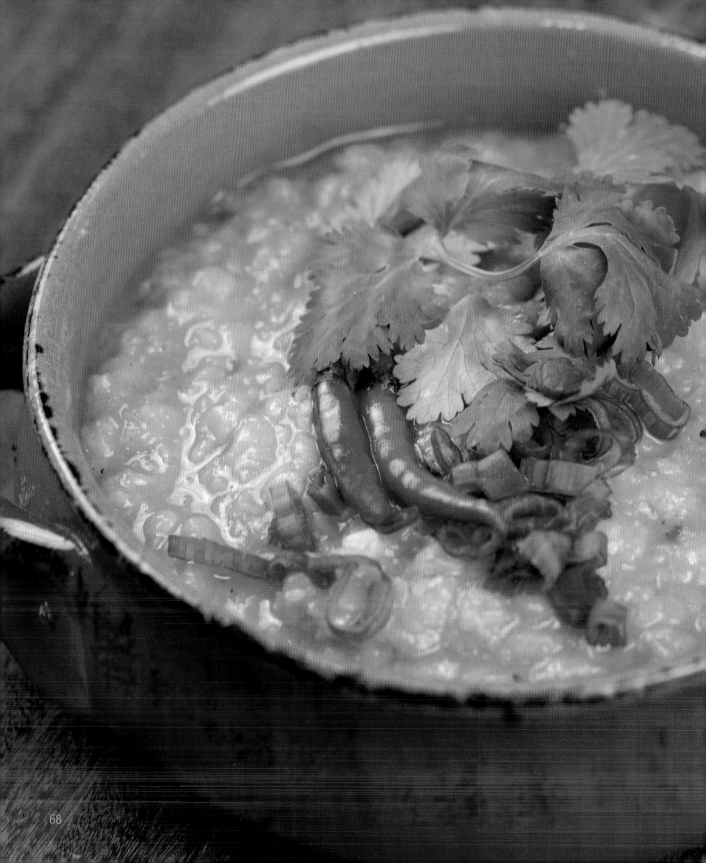

Quick and Easy LENTIL SOUP

MAKES 8 CUPS, 6 SERVINGS

Orange lentils, which cook very quickly, are the bedrock of this fundamental soup. Don't skip the garnishes, as they add vital nutrition along with great taste and visual appeal.

6 **garlic cloves,** peeled and crushed

1 teaspoon **cumin seeds**

1 teaspoon **salt**

½ teaspoon **ground turmeric**

¼ teaspoon **cayenne**

12 ounces (1½ cups) dried **orange lentils,** rinsed and drained

4 cups **water**

1 tablespoon freshly squeezed **lemon** or **lime juice**

1 tablespoon finely chopped **scallions,** for garnish

1 tablespoon finely chopped **fresh cilantro,** for garnish

1. Warm a medium saucepan over medium heat for 3 minutes.

2. Lightly mist the surface of the pan with canola oil spray.

3. Put the garlic and cumin seeds in the pan and cook, stirring frequently, until golden brown, about 3 minutes.

4. Add the salt, turmeric, and cayenne and stir to combine. Cook for 30 seconds.

5. Add the lentils and stir to coat with the spices. Add the water, cover, and bring to a boil over medium-high heat.

6. Uncover, decrease the heat to medium, and simmer until the lentils are soft, about 10 minutes.

7. If the soup is very thick, add water in ½-cup increments until it has thinned slightly. If the soup is watery, increase the heat and simmer until it has thickened slightly.

8. Remove from the heat and stir in the lemon juice.

9. Garnish with the scallions and cilantro just before serving.

Stored in an airtight container, the soup will keep in the refrigerator for about 4 days or in the freezer for about 6 weeks.

Lentil Soup WITH BUTTERNUT SQUASH AND CARROTS

MAKES 8 CUPS, 6 SERVINGS

Colorful orange lentils join vibrant butternut squash and carrots in this lovely light soup. Spoon it over brown rice or bulgur for heartier fare, or ladle it into a bowl and serve toasted bread on the side.

16 ounces (1 pound) dried **orange lentils,** rinsed and drained

8 cups **water,** plus more as needed

3 cups shredded **carrots**

3 cups frozen chopped **butternut squash**

1½ teaspoons **ground cumin**

1½ teaspoons **salt**

1 teaspoon **curry powder**

2 tablespoons finely chopped **cilantro,** for garnish

Freshly squeezed **lemon** or **lime juice,** for garnish

1 Put the lentils in a large saucepan. Add the water, carrots, squash, cumin, salt, and curry powder and bring to a boil over medium-high heat. Decrease the heat to medium and simmer, stirring occasionally, until the lentils and squash are soft, about 15 minutes.

2 If the soup is very thick, add water in ½-cup increments until it has thinned slightly. If the soup is watery, increase the heat and simmer until it has thickened slightly.

3 Garnish with the cilantro and lemon juice to taste just before serving.

Stored in an airtight container, the soup will keep in the refrigerator for about 4 days or in the freezer for about 6 weeks.

Italian BROWN LENTIL SOUP WITH VEGETABLES

MAKES 8 CUPS, 6 SERVINGS

Craving something warm and comforting? This humble soup will hit the spot. Serve it with toasted baguette slices.

16 ounces (1 pound) dried **brown lentils**, rinsed and drained

10 cups **water,** plus more as needed

2 cups shredded **carrots**

1 cup finely chopped **celery**

4 **bay leaves**

1 tablespoon **garlic granules**

1½ teaspoons **salt**

1 teaspoon **dried oregano**

Freshly squeezed **lemon** or **lime juice**

1 Put the lentils in a large saucepan. Add the water, carrots, celery, bay leaves, garlic granules, salt, and oregano and stir to combine. Bring to a boil over medium-high heat. Decrease the heat to medium and simmer until the lentils are soft, about 20 minutes.

2 If the soup is very thick, add water in ½-cup increments until it has thinned slightly. If the soup is watery, increase the heat and simmer until it has thickened slightly.

3 Add lemon juice to taste just before serving.

Stored in an airtight container, the soup will keep in the refrigerator for about 4 days or in the freezer for about 6 weeks.

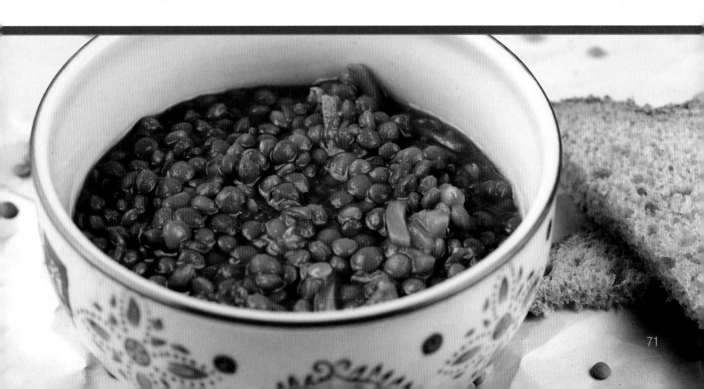

Asian NOODLE SOUP

Traditional Chinese noodle soup is considered a comfort food. It is celebrated throughout China and is always served piping hot. This soothing version is made with a homemade broth and is loaded with veggies and tofu.

1 (8-ounce) package **brown rice noodles**

½ teaspoon **canola** or **vegetable oil**

1 tablespoon crushed **garlic**

1 teaspoon grated **fresh ginger**

2 tablespoons unsalted **tomato paste**

7 cups **water**

3 tablespoons **agave nectar**

1½ teaspoons **salt**

¼ teaspoon **cayenne**

5 cups **broccoli florets**

½ cup frozen **corn kernels**

½ cup frozen **peas**

2 cups finely chopped **firm** or **extra-firm tofu**

3 tablespoons **rice vinegar**

2 tablespoons finely chopped **fresh cilantro,** for garnish

2 tablespoons finely chopped **scallions,** for garnish

1. Cook the noodles according to the package instructions and set aside.

2. Warm the oil in a large saucepan over medium heat for 2 minutes.

3. Add the garlic and ginger and cook, stirring frequently, until the garlic is golden brown, about 3 minutes. Stir in the tomato paste and 1 cup of the water and cook for 3 minutes.

4. Add the remaining water, agave nectar, salt, and cayenne and bring to a boil over high heat.

5. Decrease the heat to medium-high, add the broccoli, corn, and peas, and simmer until the broccoli is tender-crisp, about 4 minutes.

6. Stir in the tofu and remove from the heat. Stir in the vinegar.

7. For each serving, put ½ cup of the noodles into a soup bowl. Pour 1½ cups of the vegetable soup over the noodles.

8. Garnish with the cilantro and scallions just before serving.

Stored in separate airtight containers in the refrigerator, the noodles and soup will each keep for about 4 days.

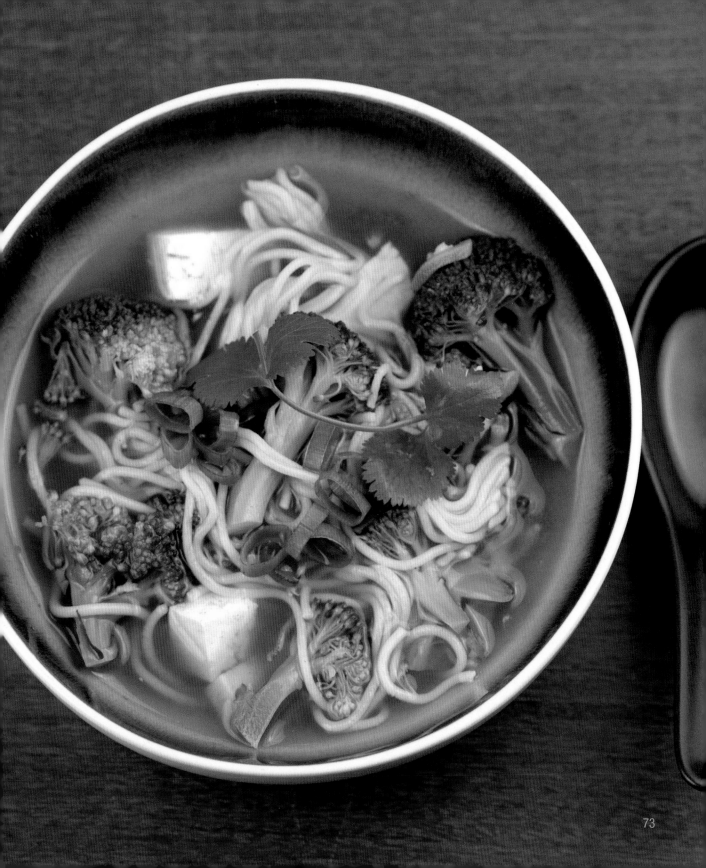

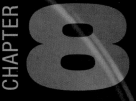

8

Sauces and Dressings

Hummus Dressing

NO-CHEESE Alfredo Sauce

Silken tofu and nutritional yeast achieve pitch-perfect harmony in this luscious, plant-based cheese sauce that is surprisingly low in fat. Spoon it liberally over pasta. For an extra-special entrée, top the pasta with Garlic Mushrooms (page 102).

½ teaspoon **olive oil**

2 cups chopped **white onions**

1 tablespoon crushed **garlic**

1 (16-ounce) package **silken tofu,** drained

¼ cup **nutritional yeast flakes**

2 tablespoons freshly squeezed **lemon juice**

1½ teaspoons **salt**

1. Put the oil in a medium skillet and warm over medium heat for 90 seconds.

2. Add the onions and garlic and stir to combine. Cook, stirring frequently, until golden brown, about 5 minutes.

3. Transfer the onion mixture to a blender. Add the tofu, nutritional yeast, lemon juice, and salt and process until smooth.

4. Pour into a medium saucepan and heat over medium-low until warm, about 5 minutes.

Stored in an airtight container, the sauce will keep in the refrigerator for about 4 days.

Marinara SAUCE

This straightforward sauce has only four ingredients and is a cinch to prepare. Plus, it can be on the table in under twenty minutes. It's an essential component of Pasta with Spinach and Chickpeas (page 100) and Veggie Lasagna (page 115).

2½ pounds **tomatoes** or **Roma tomatoes,** chopped

8 **garlic cloves,** peeled

1 tablespoon **olive oil**

¾ teaspoon **salt**

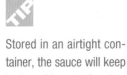

Stored in an airtight container, the sauce will keep in the refrigerator for about 4 days or in the freezer for about 6 weeks.

1 Put all the ingredients in a high-speed blender or food processor and pulse until slightly chunky.

2 Pour into a medium saucepan and cook over medium heat, stirring occasionally, until the sauce turns dark red, about 12 minutes.

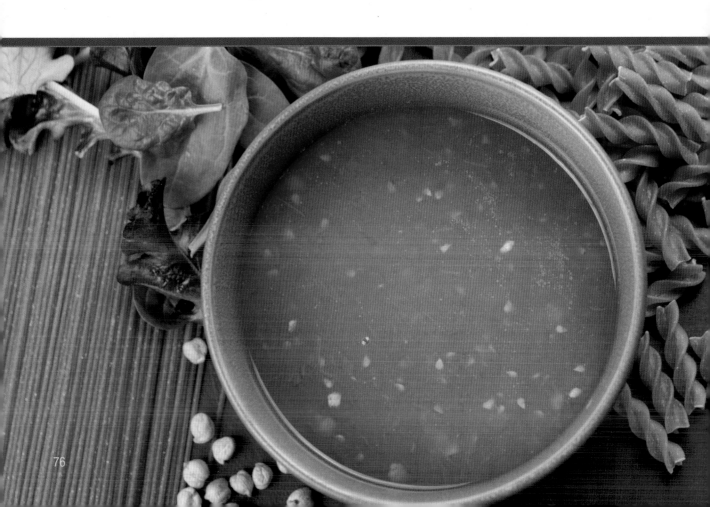

Ten-Minute PASTA SAUCE

MAKES 3 CUPS, 6 SERVINGS

Dinner will be effortless when this speedy sauce is on the menu. Toss it with your choice of pasta and veggies or use it to make Veggie Lasagna (page 115).

1 (28-ounce) can no-salt-added **crushed tomatoes**

1 tablespoon **sugar**

2 teaspoons **garlic granules**

2 teaspoons **Italian seasoning**

1 teaspoon **salt**

1 teaspoon **olive oil**

¼ teaspoon crushed **red chile flakes**

1 Put all the ingredients in a medium saucepan and stir to combine.

2 Cover and cook over medium heat for 9 minutes, stirring frequently to prevent the sauce from sticking to the bottom of the pan.

Stored in an airtight container, the sauce will keep in the refrigerator for 4 days or in the freezer for 2 weeks.

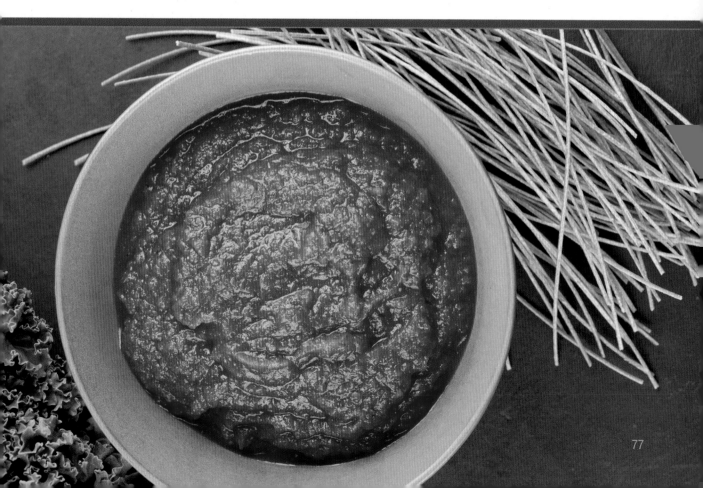

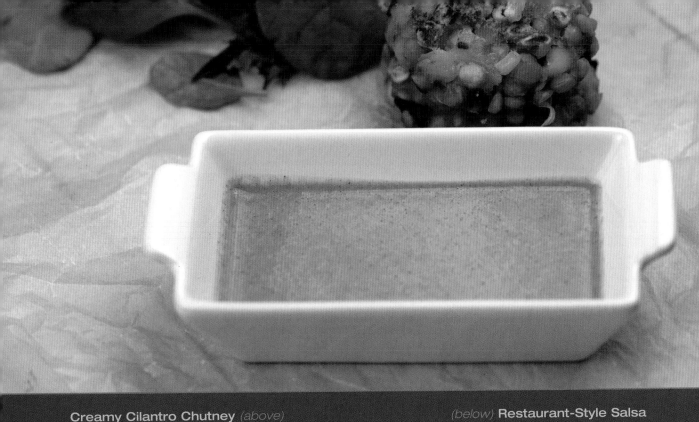

Creamy Cilantro Chutney *(above)*

(below) **Restaurant-Style Salsa**

Creamy **CILANTRO CHUTNEY**

MAKES 1½ CUPS, 6 SERVINGS

This savory, all-purpose condiment will become a staple in your kitchen. It's spectacular with Chipotle Black Bean Burgers (page 85), Yellow Split Pea Veggie Burgers (page 87), Cauliflower Wings (page 116), Baked Veggie Pakoras (page 121), and Chickpea Crêpes (page 122).

1 bunch **cilantro**

½ cup unsweetened plain **almond yogurt**

¼ cup **water**

2 tablespoons unsalted roasted **peanuts**

1½ tablespoons **agave nectar**

1½ tablespoons freshly squeezed **lemon** or **lime juice**

½ teaspoon **salt**

¼ teaspoon grated **fresh ginger**

1 Rinse the cilantro and pat it dry.

2 Put the cilantro, yogurt, water, peanuts, agave nectar, lemon juice, salt, and ginger in a blender or food processor and process until smooth.

Stored in an airtight container in the refrigerator, the chutney will keep for about 4 days.

RESTAURANT-STYLE Salsa

MAKES 3 CUPS, 6 SERVINGS

This time-honored salsa features roasted tomatoes, onion, and garlic. It makes a star appearance in Veggie Chili (page 60) and Mexican Casserole (page 128).

2 pounds ripe **tomatoes**

1 **white onion,** peeled

1 **garlic bulb,** unpeeled

½ teaspoon **salt**

½ teaspoon **chipotle chile powder**

1 Preheat the oven to 450 degrees F. Line a large baking pan with aluminum foil.

2 Put the tomatoes, onion, and garlic in the lined pan and bake for 45 minutes.

3 Remove from the oven and let cool for 20 minutes.

4 Peel the garlic cloves.

5 Put the tomatoes, onion, and garlic in a high-speed blender or food processor.

6 Add the salt and chile powder and pulse until slightly chunky.

Stored in an airtight container in the refrigerator, the salsa will keep for about 4 days.

Low-Fat CREAMY SALAD DRESSING

No one would guess that this thick, rich-tasting dressing is low in fat. Use it to top Hearty Salad (page 42), Falafel Pita Pockets (page 90), or a crisp salad mix.

1 cup unsalted cooked or canned **chickpeas**, rinsed and drained

1 cup unsweetened **soy milk**

¼ cup **nutritional yeast flakes**

¼ cup freshly squeezed **lemon** or **lime juice**

2 tablespoons raw **cashews**, soaked in water for 4 hours and drained (see tip)

1½ tablespoons **maple syrup**

1 tablespoon **capers**, drained

2 **garlic cloves**, peeled

1 teaspoon **salt**

If you use a high-speed blender to process the dressing, the cashews don't need to be soaked. Stored in an airtight container in the refrigerator, the dressing will keep for about 4 days.

1 Put all the ingredients in a blender or food processor and process until smooth.

2 Serve immediately or well chilled.

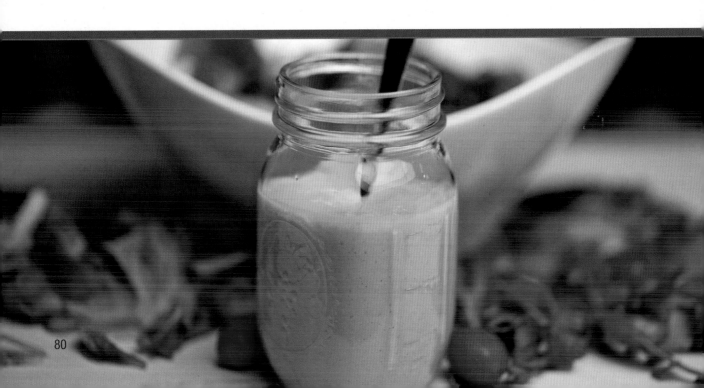

Peanut-Cilantro **SALAD DRESSING**

MAKES 1 CUP, 4 SERVINGS

The union of peanuts and cilantro makes an incomparable dressing that's phenomenal not only on salad greens but also on baked potatoes or sweet potatoes, whole grains, and legumes.

1 bunch **cilantro**

½ cup **water**

¼ cup unsalted roasted **peanuts,** or 2 tablespoons unsweetened **peanut butter**

3 tablespoons freshly squeezed **lemon** or **lime juice**

2 tablespoons **agave nectar** or **maple syrup**

2 **garlic cloves,** peeled

½ teaspoon grated **fresh ginger**

½ teaspoon **salt**

1 Rinse the cilantro and pat it dry.

2 Put the cilantro, water, peanuts, lemon juice, agave nectar, garlic, ginger, and salt in a blender or food processor and process until smooth.

3 Serve immediately or well chilled.

Stored in an airtight container in the refrigerator, the dressing will keep for about 4 days.

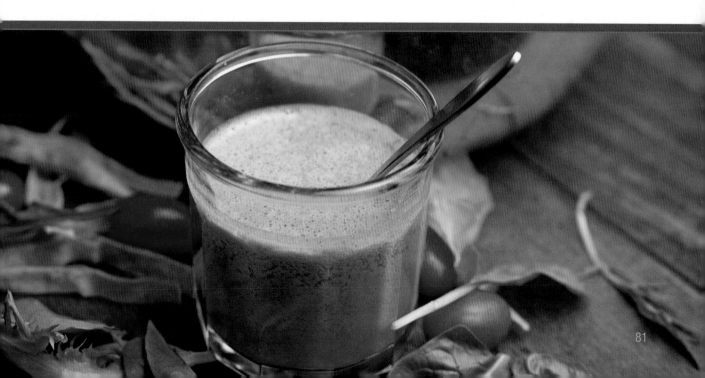

Hummus DRESSING

Chickpeas and tahini join forces to impart a creamy texture and a boost of protein to this exceptionally versatile dressing.

2 **garlic cloves,** peeled

1 cup unsalted cooked or canned **chickpeas,** rinsed and drained

1 cup **water**

2 tablespoons **tahini**

2 tablespoons freshly squeezed **lemon** or **lime juice**

½ teaspoon **salt**

Stored in an airtight container in the refrigerator, the dressing will keep for about 4 days.

1 Warm a small nonstick saucepan over medium heat for 3 minutes.

2 Lightly mist the surface of the pan with canola oil spray and roast the garlic in the pan until golden brown, 3 to 4 minutes. Turn the garlic every 1 to 2 minutes to ensure even roasting.

3 Put the garlic, chickpeas, water, tahini, lemon juice, and salt in a blender and process until smooth.

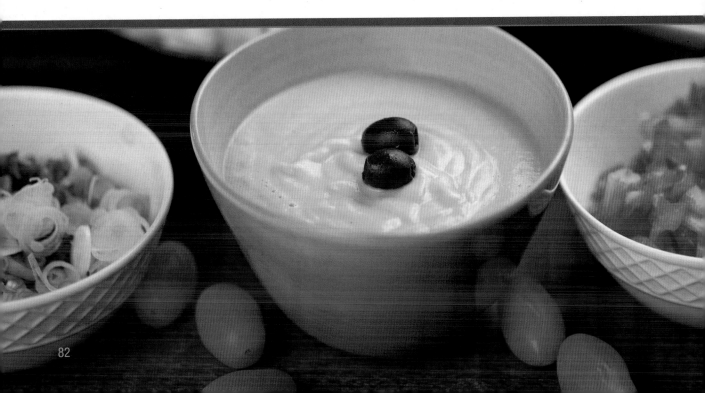

CUCUMBER Raita (SAVORY YOGURT SAUCE)

MAKES 2½ CUPS, 6 SERVINGS

Raita is a delicately seasoned yogurt dip hailing from India. Its cool, nuanced taste helps balance the peppery spices used in many Indian dishes.

½ teaspoon **cumin seeds**

1¼ cups unsweetened plain **soy, almond,** or **cashew yogurt**

1¼ cups peeled and coarsely shredded **cucumber**

¼ teaspoon **salt,** plus more as needed

1. Warm a small nonstick skillet over medium heat for 2 minutes.

2. Put the cumin seeds in the skillet and cook, stirring frequently, until fragrant and golden brown, about 2 minutes. Remove from the heat.

3. Put the yogurt, cucumber, and salt in a medium bowl and stir until well combined. Add more salt to taste, if desired.

4. Sprinkle the toasted cumin seeds over the top. Serve well chilled.

Stored in an airtight container in the refrigerator, the raita will keep for about 4 days.

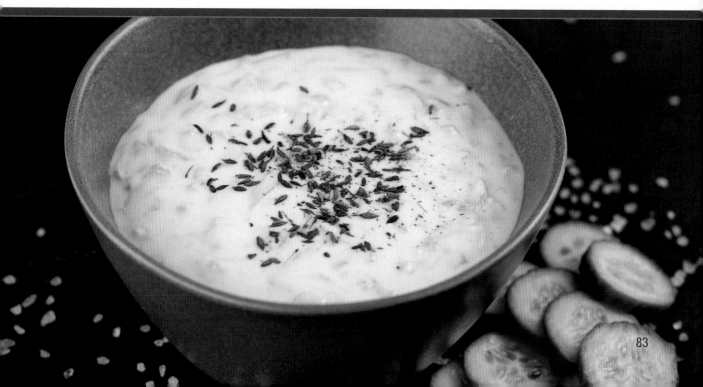

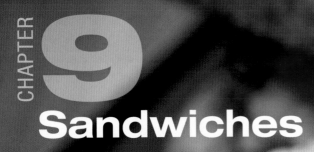

Sandwiches

Chickpea Tuna Salad Sandwich

Chipotle BLACK BEAN BURGERS

MAKES 6 BURGERS

Black beans and sweet potato are the framework for these firm, succulent burgers. Showcase them on whole-grain burger buns with all the trimmings.

1 large **sweet potato,** unpeeled

1 (15-ounce) can unsalted **black beans,** rinsed and drained

1 cup finely chopped **red onion**

½ cup finely chopped **fresh cilantro,** lightly packed

¾ teaspoon **chipotle chile powder**

½ teaspoon **salt**

1. Preheat the oven to 400 degrees F. Line a small baking pan with parchment paper.

2. Lay the sweet potato in the lined pan and bake for 40 minutes, until a fork can be easily inserted into the center. Let cool for 15 minutes, then coarsely chop.

3. Put the sweet potato and beans in a large bowl and mash with a potato masher or the back of a sturdy large fork until slightly chunky.

4. Add the onion, cilantro, chile powder, and salt and stir until well combined.

5. Using your hands, form the mixture into 6 flat burger patties.

6. Warm a large nonstick skillet over medium heat for 3 minutes.

7. Lightly mist the skillet with canola oil spray.

8. Cook the patties in the skillet until golden brown all over, 3 to 4 minutes per side.

Stored in an airtight container in the refrigerator, the uncooked or cooked burger patties will keep for about 4 days.

NAVY BEAN AND KALE Burgers

MAKES 6 BURGERS

Buttery navy beans and crunchy kale are combined with smoked paprika to create these unique burgers. Prep takes merely ten minutes, so they are ideal to make for dinner on busy days. Serve them on whole-grain burger buns with all the fixin's: tomatoes, onion, lettuce, and ketchup or Creamy Cilantro Chutney (page 79).

2 (15-ounce) cans unsalted **navy beans,** rinsed and drained

1 cup finely chopped **kale,** firmly packed

½ cup finely chopped **scallions**

2 teaspoons **smoked paprika**

2 teaspoons **garlic granules**

¾ teaspoon **salt**

1. Put the beans in a large bowl and mash with a potato masher or the back of a sturdy large fork until slightly chunky.

2. Add the kale, scallions, paprika, garlic granules, and salt and stir until well combined.

3. Using your hands, form the mixture into 6 flat burger patties.

4. Warm a large nonstick skillet over medium heat for 3 minutes.

5. Lightly mist the skillet with canola oil spray.

6. Cook the patties in the skillet until golden brown all over, 3 to 4 minutes per side.

Stored in an airtight container in the refrigerator, the uncooked or cooked burger patties will keep for about 4 days.

Yellow Split Pea VEGGIE BURGERS

MAKES 10 SMALL BURGERS

Yellow split peas and potatoes are infused with golden turmeric to create eye-catching burgers that are packed with protein, fiber, and antioxidants. Serve them with ketchup or Creamy Cilantro Chutney (page 79).

1 pound **potatoes,** unpeeled

6 ounces (¾ cup) dried **yellow split peas,** rinsed and drained

¼ white **onion,** finely chopped

½ teaspoon **salt**

½ teaspoon **cayenne**

½ teaspoon **ground turmeric**

1. Put the potatoes in a medium saucepan and add enough water to cover them completely. Bring to a boil over medium-high heat. Decrease the heat to medium and simmer until the potatoes are soft, about 35 minutes. Drain and rinse with cold water.

2. Put the split peas in a small saucepan and cover with water. Bring to a boil over medium-high heat. Decrease the heat to medium and simmer, stirring occasionally, until soft, about 30 minutes. Drain and rinse with cold water.

3. Put the potatoes in a large bowl and mash with a potato masher or the back of a sturdy large fork until slightly chunky.

4. Add the split peas, onion, salt, cayenne, and turmeric and stir until evenly distributed.

5. Using your hands, form the mixture into 10 flat burger patties.

6. Warm a large nonstick skillet over medium heat for 3 minutes.

7. Lightly mist the skillet with canola oil spray. Cook the patties in the skillet until golden brown all over, 3 to 4 minutes per side.

8. Cook the patties in the skillet until golden brown all over, 3 to 4 minutes per side.

Stored in an airtight container in the refrigerator, the uncooked or cooked burger patties will keep for about 4 days.

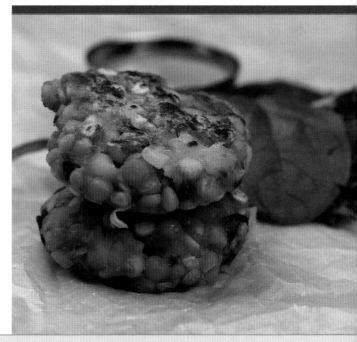

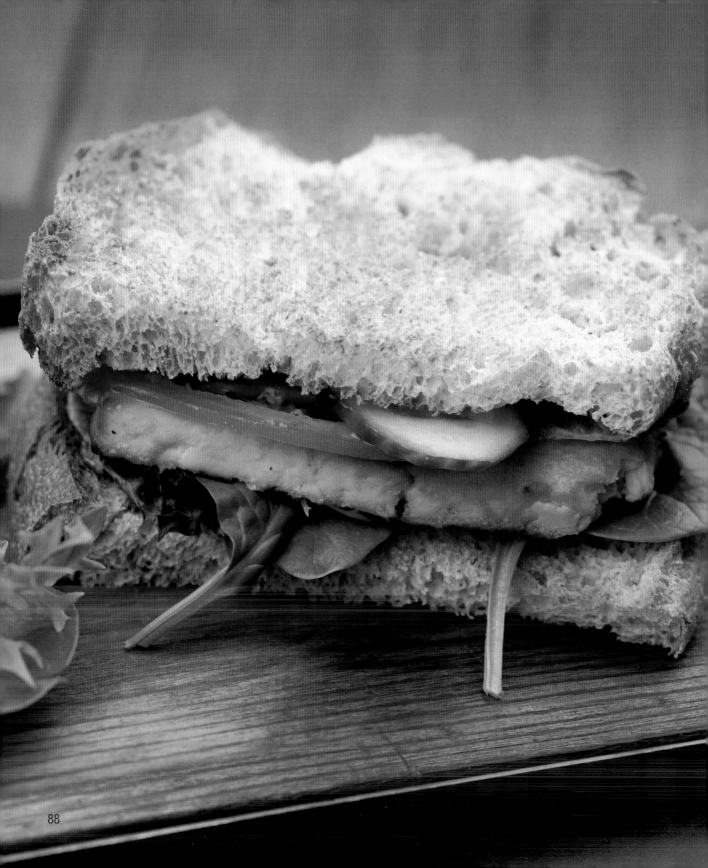

Grilled TOFU SANDWICHES

MAKES 4 SANDWICHES

Tofu is marinated, then grilled to perfection for these fabulous open-faced sandwiches. Enjoy them for lunch or dinner.

1 cup unsalted cooked or canned **chickpeas,** rinsed and drained

1 cup unsweetened plain **soy** or **almond milk**

3 tablespoons low-sodium **soy sauce**

3 tablespoons freshly squeezed **lemon** or **lime juice**

1½ tablespoons **maple syrup**

¾ teaspoon grated **fresh ginger**

2 **garlic cloves,** peeled

1 (14-ounce) package **firm** or **extra-firm tofu**

4 slices **whole wheat bread,** toasted

Salad greens

Sliced **tomato**

Sliced **cucumber**

1. To make the marinade, put the chickpeas, milk, soy sauce, lemon juice, maple syrup, ginger, and garlic in a blender and process until smooth.

2. Drain the tofu and slice it into 8 rectangular pieces.

3. Put the tofu in a large storage container and cover completely with the marinade. Seal tightly and refrigerate for 4 to 8 hours.

4. Remove the tofu from the marinade and set the marinade aside. Cook the tofu in an air fryer on high until golden brown, about 10 minutes. Alternatively, lightly mist a nonstick skillet with canola oil spray and cook the tofu over medium heat until golden brown, about 5 minutes per side.

5. Spread some of the reserved marinate over the tofu. Arrange the tofu on the toasted bread and top with salad greens, tomato, and cucumber to taste.

Stored in an airtight container in the refrigerator, the uncooked or cooked tofu slices will keep for about 3 days.

Falafel PITA POCKETS

Falafels are traditionally fried in oil, which turns an otherwise healthy food into a high-fat fiasco. These falafels, however, are baked, not fried, so they are low in fat yet incredibly delicious.

4 cups unsalted cooked or canned **chickpeas,** rinsed and drained

½ cup finely chopped **white** or **red onion**

¼ cup finely chopped **Italian parsley,** lightly packed

1½ teaspoons **garlic granules**

1 teaspoon **ground cumin**

½ teaspoon **dried basil**

½ teaspoon **salt**

1 cup **Hummus Dressing** (page 82)

4 **whole wheat pita rounds,** toasted

Salad greens

Finely chopped **tomato**

Finely chopped **cucumber**

1 Preheat the oven to 400 degrees F. Line a large baking sheet with parchment paper.

2 Put the chickpeas in a large bowl and mash them with a potato masher or the back of a sturdy large fork until mushy.

3 Add the onion, parsley, garlic granules, cumin, basil, and salt and stir until well combined.

4 Form the mixture into 16 balls, about 1½ inches in diameter.

5 Arrange the balls on the lined baking sheet and bake for 25 to 30 minutes, until the exterior is slightly crispy.

6 Just before serving, fill the pocket of each pita round with 2 falafels and drizzle ¼ cup of the dressing over them. Add salad greens, tomato, and cucumber to taste.

Stored in an airtight container in the refrigerator, the uncooked or cooked falafels will keep for about 4 days.

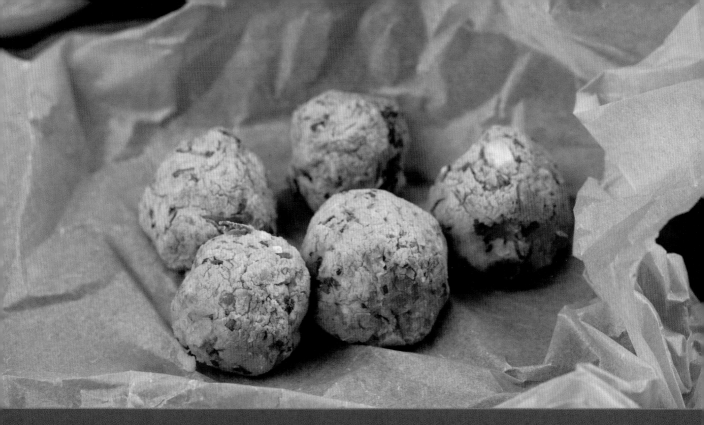

Falafel Pita Pockets *(above)*   *(below)* **Cauliflower Panini**

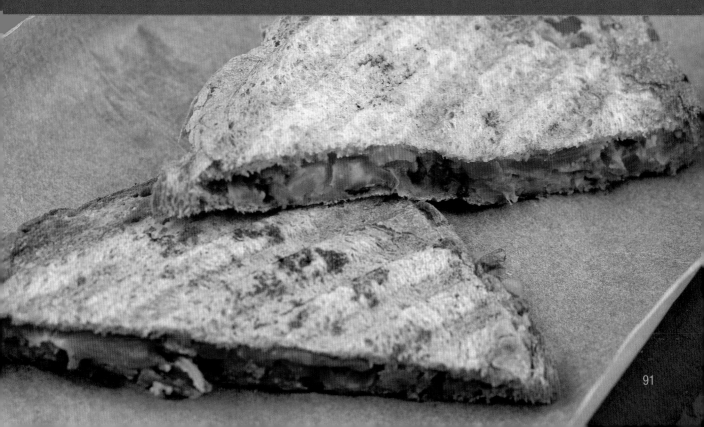

CAULIFLOWER Panini

Fresh herbs and pert spices add pizzazz to mashed cauliflower, turning it into a scrumptious filling for a panini. Serve it with Creamy Cilantro Chutney (page 79) or ketchup.

1 **cauliflower,** chopped

1 **red** or **yellow onion,** finely chopped

1 teaspoon **cumin seeds**

¾ teaspoon **salt**

½ teaspoon **ground turmeric**

¼ teaspoon **cayenne**

¼ cup finely chopped **fresh cilantro,** lightly packed

8 slices **whole wheat bread**

1 **tomato,** thinly sliced

1. Put the cauliflower in a medium saucepan. Add enough water to cover the cauliflower completely and bring to a boil over medium-high heat. Decrease the heat to medium and simmer until the cauliflower is very soft, about 20 minutes. Remove from the heat and drain.

2. Warm a medium saucepan over medium-high heat for 3 minutes.

3. Lightly mist the surface of the pan with canola oil spray.

4. Put the onion in the pan and cook, stirring frequently, until golden brown, about 3 minutes.

5. Add the cumin seeds, salt, turmeric, and cayenne and cook, stirring frequently, until the cumin seeds are golden brown, about 2 minutes. Remove from the heat.

6. Add the cauliflower and cilantro and stir until evenly combined.

7. Warm a small nonstick skillet over medium heat for 3 minutes.

8. For each sandwich, spread a thick layer of the cauliflower mixture on one slice of bread. Top with tomato slices and another slice of bread.

9. Cook in the skillet until golden brown all over, about 3 minutes per side. Alternatively, grill the sandwich in a panini press on medium-high heat until golden brown, about 4 minutes.

Stored in an airtight container in the refrigerator, the cauliflower filling will keep for about 3 days.

CHICKPEA Tuna Salad SANDWICHES

MAKES 4 SERVINGS

The combination of chickpeas, mayo, and mustard creates a tangy salad that is superb when scooped atop crisp lettuce leaves or stuffed into whole-grain pita pockets.

3 (15-ounce) cans unsalted **chickpeas,** rinsed and drained

1½ cups finely chopped **celery**

1 cup shredded **carrots**

½ cup finely chopped **scallions** or **white onion**

½ cup **sweet pickle relish**

⅓ cup low-fat **vegan mayonnaise**

1½ tablespoons stone-ground **mustard**

½ teaspoon **salt**

¼ teaspoon ground **black pepper**

4 **whole wheat pita rounds,** or 4 slices **whole wheat bread,** toasted

Salad greens

Sliced **tomatoes**

1   Put the chickpeas in a large bowl and mash them well with a potato masher or the back of a sturdy large fork.

2   Add the celery, carrots, scallions, relish, mayonnaise, mustard, salt, and pepper and stir until well combined.

3   To serve, spoon the chickpea salad into the pocket of each pita round and top with salad greens and tomatoes to taste.

Stored in an airtight container in the refrigerator, the chickpea salad will keep for 2 to 3 days.

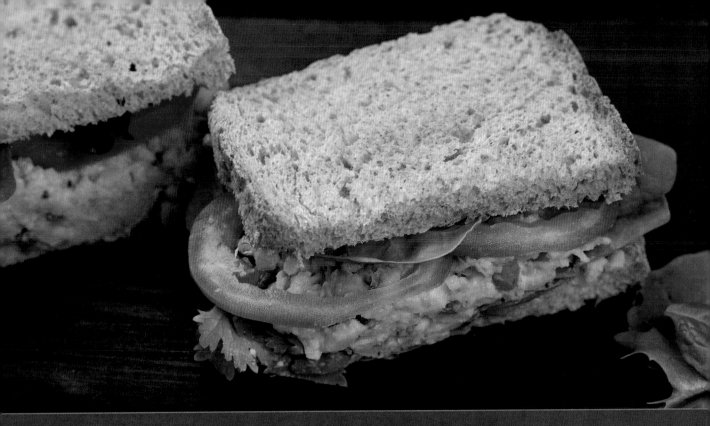

Chickpea Tuna Salad Sandwiches *(above)*

(below) **Potato Panini**

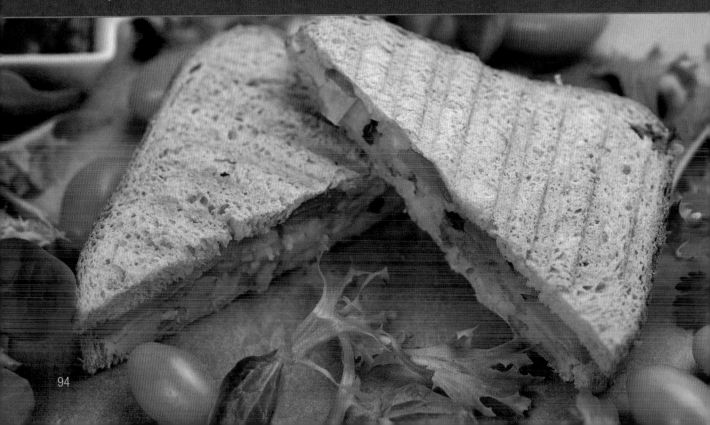

94

POTATO Panini

Mashed potatoes, onion, and cilantro form a trifecta of flavor in this substantial panini. Serve it warm, accompanied by Creamy Cilantro Chutney (page 79) or ketchup.

4 **red** or **white potatoes**

½ **white onion,** finely chopped

2 tablespoons finely chopped **fresh cilantro**

½ teaspoon **salt**

¼ teaspoon **cayenne** or crushed **red chile flakes**

8 slices **whole wheat bread**

1 **tomato,** thinly sliced

1. Put the potatoes in a medium saucepan. Add enough water to cover the potatoes completely and bring to a boil over medium-high heat. Decrease the heat to medium and simmer until the potatoes are very soft, about 40 minutes.

2. Remove from the heat and drain. Let cool for 15 minutes.

3. Put the potatoes in a large bowl and mash with a potato masher or the back of a sturdy large fork until slightly lumpy.

4. Add the onion, cilantro, salt, and cayenne and stir until evenly distributed.

5. Warm a small nonstick skillet over medium heat for 3 minutes.

6. For each sandwich, spread a thick layer of the potato mixture on one slice of bread. Top with tomato slices and another slice of bread.

7. Cook in the skillet until golden brown all over, about 3 minutes per side. Alternatively, grill the sandwich in a panini press on medium-high heat until golden brown, about 4 minutes.

Stored in an airtight container in the refrigerator, the potato filling will keep for about 3 days.

MAKES 6 SERVINGS

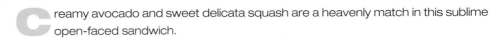

Creamy avocado and sweet delicata squash are a heavenly match in this sublime open-faced sandwich.

1 small **delicata squash**

1 **avocado**

6 slices **whole wheat bread,** toasted

Salt

Ground **black pepper**

Garlic granules

1 Preheat the oven to 400 degrees F. Line a small baking pan with parchment paper.

2 Lay the squash in the lined pan and bake for 20 minutes, until a fork can be easily inserted into the center. Let cool for 20 minutes.

3 Slice the squash into ½-inch-thick rings. Remove the skin from each ring and scoop out the seeds with a spoon. Discard the skin and seeds.

4 Scoop out the avocado pulp with a spoon and put it into a small bowl. Mash the pulp with the back of a sturdy fork.

5 For each sandwich, spread a thin layer of the avocado over a slice of the toasted bread. Top with a portion of the squash.

6 Sprinkle with salt, pepper, and garlic granules to taste.

Stored in separate airtight containers in the refrigerator, the avocado will keep for about 2 days and the squash for about 4 days.

Hummus SANDWICHES

If you have Roasted Garlic Hummus premade, these open-faced sandwiches will take mere minutes to assemble. They offer a power-packed punch of protein, fiber, and deliciousness.

¾ cup **Roasted Garlic Hummus** (page 50)

4 slices **whole wheat bread,** toasted

1 **tomato,** thinly sliced

½ **cucumber,** thinly sliced

Salt

Ground **black pepper**

1. For each sandwich, spread a thick layer of the hummus over a slice of the toasted bread.

2. Top with a portion of the tomato and cucumber slices.

3. Sprinkle with salt and pepper to taste. Serve immediately.

MUSHROOM Toast

Just one bite of this deceptively simple dish will have your taste buds extolling the unexpected alliance of garlicky mushrooms and hummus.

¾ cup **Edamame Hummus** (page 51)

4 slices **whole wheat bread,** toasted

2½ cups **Garlic Mushrooms** (page 102)

Crushed **red chile flakes**

1. For each serving, spread a thick layer of the hummus over a sliced of the toasted bread.

2. Top with a portion of the mushrooms.

3. Sprinkle with chile flakes to taste. Serve immediately.

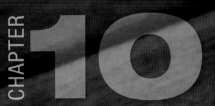

Tofu Curry

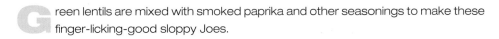

Lentil SLOPPY JOES

MAKES 3 CUPS, 4 SERVINGS

Green lentils are mixed with smoked paprika and other seasonings to make these finger-licking-good sloppy Joes.

½ teaspoon **olive oil**

½ **yellow onion,** finely chopped

3 **garlic cloves,** peeled and crushed

2 tablespoons unsalted **tomato paste**

10 ounces (1¼ cups) dried **green lentils,** rinsed and drained

4¼ cups **water,** plus more as needed

2 tablespoons **maple syrup**

1 tablespoon **apple cider vinegar**

1½ teaspoons **smoked paprika**

¾ teaspoon **salt**

4 **whole wheat pita rounds,** toasted

1 cup finely chopped **lettuce,** lightly packed

½ cup finely chopped **tomato**

½ cup finely chopped **cucumber**

1. Put the oil in a large saucepan and warm over medium heat for 2 minutes.

2. Add the onion and cook, stirring frequently, until golden brown, about 3 minutes.

3. Add the garlic and cook, stirring frequently, until golden brown, about 2 minutes.

4. Add the tomato paste and stir until well combined.

5. Add the lentils, water, maple syrup, vinegar, paprika, and salt and stir until well combined. Bring to a boil over medium-high heat. Decrease the heat to medium and simmer until the lentils are soft, about 45 minutes.

6. If the sauce is very thick, add water in ½-cup increments until it has thinned slightly. If the sauce is watery, increase the heat and simmer until it has thickened slightly.

7. Fill the pocket of each pita round with about ½ cup of the sloppy Joe mixture.

8. Top with lettuce, tomato, and cucumber and serve immediately.

Stored in an airtight container, the lentils will keep in the refrigerator for about 4 days or in the freezer for about 6 weeks.

Fettuccine **ALFREDO** WITH MUSHROOMS

MAKES 4 SERVINGS

This dish is sure to satisfy the craving for a creamy pasta meal. The mushrooms add texture and heartiness.

If the sauce and mushrooms were premade, warm them separately in the microwave or on the stove top before using. Stored in separate airtight containers in the refrigerator, the fettuccine, sauce, and mushrooms will each keep for about 4 days.

8 ounces **whole wheat fettuccine, spaghetti, or linguine**

3½ cups **No-Cheese Alfredo Sauce** (page 75; see tip)

2½ cups **Garlic Mushrooms** (page 102; see tip)

2 tablespoons finely chopped **Italian parsley,** for garnish

Crushed **red chile flakes,** for garnish

1 Cook the fettuccine according to the package instructions.

2 Spoon the sauce over the fettuccine and top with the mushrooms.

3 Garnish with the parsley just before serving. Sprinkle with chile flakes to taste.

Pasta **WITH SPINACH AND CHICKPEAS**

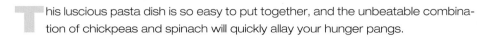

MAKES 4 SERVINGS

This luscious pasta dish is so easy to put together, and the unbeatable combination of chickpeas and spinach will quickly allay your hunger pangs.

8 ounces **whole wheat fettuccine, spaghetti, or linguine**

3½ cups **Marinara Sauce** (page 76) or **Ten-Minute Pasta Sauce** (page 77)

1 (5-ounce) package **baby spinach**

1 (15-ounce) can unsalted **chickpeas,** rinsed and drained

12 pitted **kalamata olives,** for garnish

Crushed **red chile flakes,** for garnish

Stored in separate airtight containers in the refrigerator, the fettuccine and sauce will each keep for about 4 days.

1 Cook the pasta according to the package instructions and set aside.

2 Put the chickpeas, sauce, and spinach in a medium saucepan and stir to combine. Cook over medium-high heat, stirring frequently, until the spinach wilts and the sauce is hot, about 5 minutes.

3 Spoon the warm sauce over the pasta. Garnish with the olives and sprinkle with chile flakes to taste.

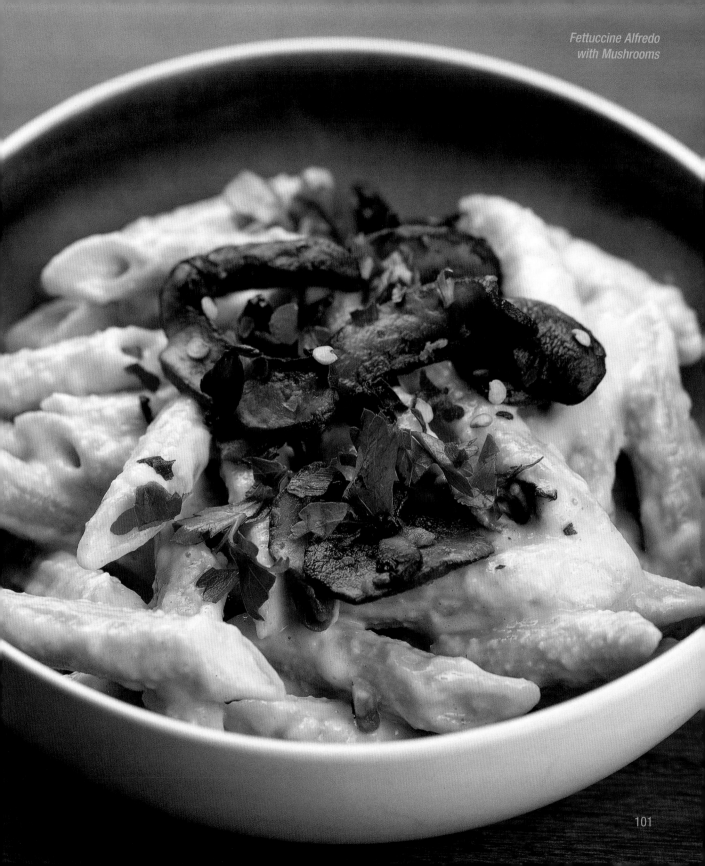

GARLIC Mushrooms

ushrooms have a pleasing hearty texture and earthy taste, which is enhanced when they are sautéed with garlic. Try these savory morsels over pasta topped with No-Cheese Alfredo Sauce (page 75) or as an accompaniment to any main dish.

1 tablespoon crushed **garlic**

1 teaspoon **olive oil**

½ teaspoon **salt**

6 cups sliced **shiitake, cremini,** or **baby bella mushrooms**

Stored in an airtight container in the refrigerator, the mushrooms will keep for about 4 days.

1 Warm a large, wide saucepan over medium heat for 3 minutes.

2 Spread the oil over the surface of the pan.

3 Add the garlic and cook, stirring frequently, until golden brown, about 2 minutes.

4 Add the mushrooms and salt and stir well to combine. The salt will cause the mushrooms to release their liquid, which will help soften and cook them.

5 Cook uncovered until the mushrooms are soft and most of the liquid has evaporated, about 12 minutes.

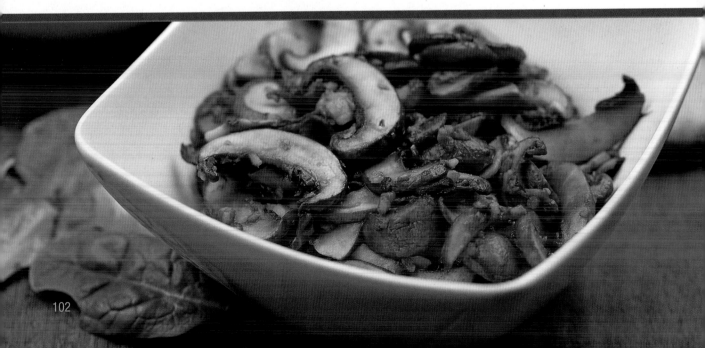

Baked BEANS

Baked beans are famous for their blend of savory, sweet, and tangy tastes, and this version is the complete package. Turn this dish into a full meal by serving it with a leafy green veggie or salad and a cooked whole grain, such as brown rice or quinoa.

16 ounces (1 pound) dried **pinto beans,** rinsed, drained, and soaked in water for 8 to 12 hours

1 teaspoon **olive oil**

1 **yellow onion,** finely chopped

8 **garlic cloves,** peeled and crushed

10 cups **water**

¼ cup unsalted **tomato paste**

¼ cup **maple syrup**

2 tablespoons **apple cider vinegar**

1 tablespoon **smoked paprika**

1½ teaspoons **salt**

1. Drain and rinse the beans and set aside.

2. Warm the oil in a large, wide saucepan over medium heat for 2 minutes.

3. Add the onion and cook, stirring frequently, until golden brown, about 4 minutes.

4. Add the garlic and cook, stirring frequently, until golden brown, about 2 minutes.

5. Add the water, tomato paste, maple syrup, vinegar, paprika, and salt and stir with a large spoon until the tomato paste is dissolved and the mixture is well combined.

6. Bring to a boil over high heat. Decrease the heat to medium-high and simmer, stirring occasionally, until the beans are soft, about 45 minutes.

7. If the sauce is very thick, add water in ½-cup increments until it has thinned slightly. If the sauce is watery, increase the heat and simmer until it has thickened slightly.

Stored in an airtight container, the beans will keep in the refrigerator for about 4 days or in the freezer for about 4 weeks.

Soba Noodles **WITH VEGETABLES**

Asian-style wheat noodles team up with bok choy and edamame to create an enticing one-dish meal that's rich in calcium and fiber.

3 tablespoons crushed **garlic**

2 cups frozen **edamame**

1½ cups **water**

1 teaspoon **salt**

2 bunches **bok choy,** finely chopped (about 6 cups, firmly packed)

1 cup shredded **carrots**

12 ounces **soba noodles**

2 tablespoons **rice vinegar**

Soy sauce, as needed

Sriracha sauce, as needed

1. Warm a large, wide saucepan over medium heat for 3 minutes.

2. Lightly mist the surface of the pan with canola oil spray.

3. Put the garlic in the pan and cook, stirring frequently, until golden brown, about 2 minutes.

4. Add the edamame, water, and salt and stir to combine. Cover and cook, stirring occasionally, until the edamame is soft, about 8 minutes.

5. Add the bok choy and carrots and stir to combine. Cover and cook, stirring occasionally, until the bok choy wilts, about 3 minutes. Remove from the heat.

6. Cook the soba noodles according to the package directions. Drain and add them to the vegetables (see tip).

7. Add the vinegar and gently stir until it is evenly distributed.

8. Add soy sauce as desired for a saltier taste and sriracha sauce as desired for a spicier taste.

TIP

Soba noodles tend to stick together, so for the best results, mix them with the vegetables immediately after cooking and draining them. Stored in an airtight container in the refrigerator, the noodles with vegetables will keep for about 4 days.

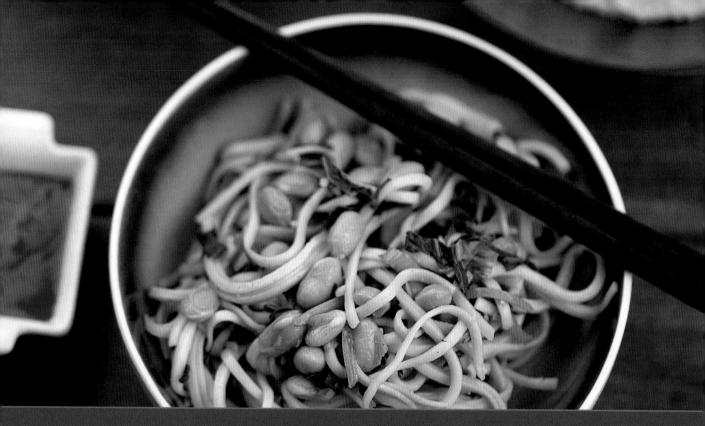

Soba Noodles with Vegetables *(above)*

(below) **Tofu Curry**

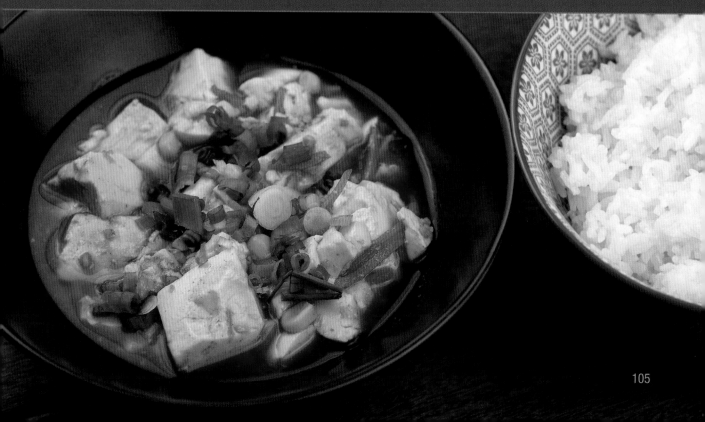

105

TOFU Curry

 ilken tofu, vegetables, and spices intermingle in this mild but lively curry. It partners perfectly with short-grain brown rice.

1 tablespoon crushed **garlic**

1 teaspoon grated **fresh ginger**

1 tablespoon unsalted **tomato paste**

¾ cup **water**

¼ cup shredded **carrots**

¼ cup frozen **corn kernels**

2 tablespoons low-sodium **soy sauce**

1 tablespoon **agave nectar**

1 tablespoon **rice vinegar**

1 teaspoon **sriracha sauce**

1 (16-ounce) package **silken tofu,** drained and cut into 1-inch cubes (see tip)

¼ cup finely chopped **scallions,** for garnish

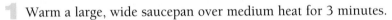

1 Warm a large, wide saucepan over medium heat for 3 minutes.

2 Lightly mist the surface of the pan with canola oil spray.

3 Put the garlic and ginger in the pan and cook, stirring frequently, until the garlic is golden brown, about 2 minutes.

4 Add the tomato paste and water and stir with a large spoon until the paste is thoroughly dissolved.

5 Add the carrots and corn and stir until well combined. Cover and cook over medium heat until the carrots are soft, about 10 minutes.

6 Add the soy sauce, agave nectar, vinegar, and sriracha sauce and stir until well combined.

7 Gently stir in the tofu. Cover and cook briefly over medium heat to let the tofu soak up some of the flavor, about 4 minutes.

8 Garnish with the scallions just before serving.

Silken tofu is very delicate and falls apart easily, so use care when you handle it. Stored in an airtight container in the refrigerator, the curry will keep for about 4 days.

Marinated TOFU STEAKS

MAKES 12 STEAKS, 6 SERVINGS

These naturally tender steaks are soft on the inside and slightly crispy on the outside. Serve them with a crisp, leafy green salad tossed with Low-Fat Creamy Salad Dressing (page 80).

2 (16-ounce) packages **firm** or **extra-firm tofu**

1¾ cups unsweetened plain **soy** or **almond milk**

¼ cup unsalted cooked or canned **chickpeas,** rinsed and drained

6 tablespoons freshly squeezed **lemon juice**

3 tablespoons **yellow mustard**

2 tablespoons **dried oregano**

4 **garlic cloves,** peeled

1 teaspoon **salt**

1 teaspoon ground **black pepper**

1 Slice each block of tofu into 6 thin rectangles. Lightly tap the sharp edge of a knife on the flat surface of each rectangle to make a crisscross pattern.

2 To make the marinade, put the milk, chickpeas, lemon juice, mustard, oregano, garlic, salt, and pepper in a blender and process until smooth. Pour the marinade into a wide storage dish.

3 Arrange the tofu rectangles in a single layer in the marinade so that all sides are covered.

4 Cover tightly and let the tofu marinate in the refrigerator for 2 hours, then carefully turn the slices over and marinate for 2 hours longer.

5 Cook the tofu in an air fryer on the high setting until golden brown, about 10 minutes. Alternatively, lightly mist a nonstick skillet with canola oil spray and cook the steaks over medium heat until golden brown, about 5 minutes per side. Serve warm.

Stored in an airtight container in the refrigerator, the uncooked or grilled tofu steaks will keep for about 3 days.

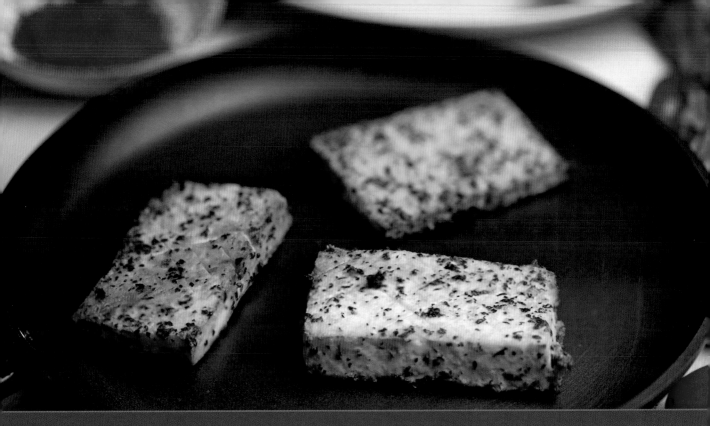

Marinated Tofu Steaks *(above)*

(below) Black Bean Quesadillas

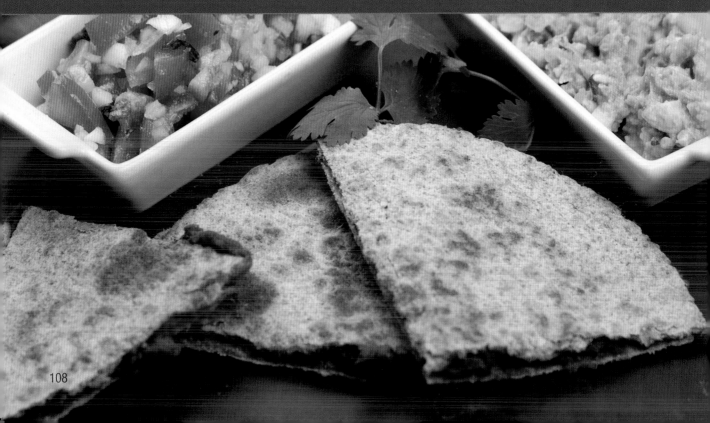

BLACK BEAN Quesadillas

Originating in Mexico, quesadillas are a type of taco made with either wheat or corn tortillas. This plant-based version is packed with protein-rich beans and zippy fresh salsa for a fiesta in your mouth.

1 **red onion,** finely chopped

2 (15-ounce) cans unsalted **black** or **pinto beans,** rinsed and drained

⅓ cup **Salsa Fresca** (page 45), plus more for serving

1 tablespoon **garlic granules**

½ teaspoon **salt**

½ teaspoon **chipotle chile powder**

8 **whole wheat tortillas**

1 cup **Classic Guacamole** (page 49), for serving

1. Warm a small saucepan over medium heat for 3 minutes.

2. Lightly mist the surface of the pan with canola oil spray.

3. Put the onion in the pan and cook over medium-high heat until golden brown, about 4 minutes. Remove from the heat.

4. Put the onion, beans, salsa, garlic granules, salt, and chile powder in a blender and process until smooth.

5. Warm a medium nonstick skillet over medium heat for 3 minutes.

6. Spread a thick layer of beans in between 2 of the tortillas to make a quesadilla. Cook each quesadilla in the hot skillet until golden brown all over, about 3 minutes per side.

7. Serve with the guacamole and additional salsa on the side.

Stored in an airtight container in the refrigerator, the beans will keep for about 4 days.

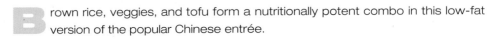

Veggie FRIED RICE

Brown rice, veggies, and tofu form a nutritionally potent combo in this low-fat version of the popular Chinese entrée.

1 (14-ounce) package **firm** or **extra-firm tofu,** drained

1½ cups **Creamy Cilantro Chutney** (page 79)

1 teaspoon **sesame oil**

2 tablespoons crushed **garlic**

1 teaspoon grated **fresh ginger**

¼ cup **water**

½ small **cabbage,** finely chopped

1 cup frozen **peas**

½ cup frozen **corn kernels**

¼ cup low-sodium **soy sauce**

2 tablespoons **sugar**

½ teaspoon **cayenne**

3 cups cooked brown **jasmine** or short-grain **brown rice**

¼ cup finely chopped **scallions,** for garnish

1. Slice the tofu into ½-inch cubes and transfer to a medium bowl. Pour the chutney over the tofu, cover tightly, and let marinate in the refrigerator for at least 6 hours.

2. Cook the tofu in an air fryer on the high setting until golden brown, about 10 minutes. Alternatively, preheat the oven on the broiler setting. Line a baking sheet with parchment paper and arrange the tofu on it in a single layer. Broil in the oven until golden brown, about 10 minutes. Set aside.

3. Warm the oil in a large, wide saucepan over medium heat for 3 minutes.

4. Put the garlic and ginger in the pan and cook, stirring frequently, until the garlic is golden brown, about 2 minutes. Add the water to prevent burning.

5. Add the cabbage, peas, and corn and stir with a large spoon until well combined. Cook over medium heat, stirring frequently, until the cabbage is slightly soft, about 5 minutes.

6. Put the soy sauce, sugar, and cayenne in a small bowl and stir until well combined.

7. Add the soy sauce mixture and rice to the vegetables and stir with a large spoon until evenly distributed. Cook uncovered, stirring frequently, until the rice is warm, about 4 minutes.

8. Transfer to a serving dish and top with the tofu.

9. Garnish with the scallions just before serving.

Stored in an airtight container in the refrigerator, the fried rice and tofu will keep for about 4 days.

Bulgur PILAF

Bulgur is combined with yellow split peas, herbs, and veggies to create a bold pilaf that is light yet satiating.

2 cups cooked **bulgur**

2 cups finely chopped **cucumbers**

1½ cups cooked **yellow split peas**

½ cup finely chopped **white onion**

¼ cup pitted **kalamata olives**

¼ cup finely chopped **Italian parsley**, lightly packed

1½ tablespoons **white wine vinegar**

1 tablespoon finely chopped **fresh mint**

½ teaspoon **salt**

1 teaspoon **garlic granules**

¼ teaspoon **cayenne**

¼ teaspoon **dried dill weed**

1 Put all the ingredients in a large bowl and stir until well combined.

2 Serve at room temperature.

Stored in an airtight container in the refrigerator, the pilaf will keep for about 4 days.

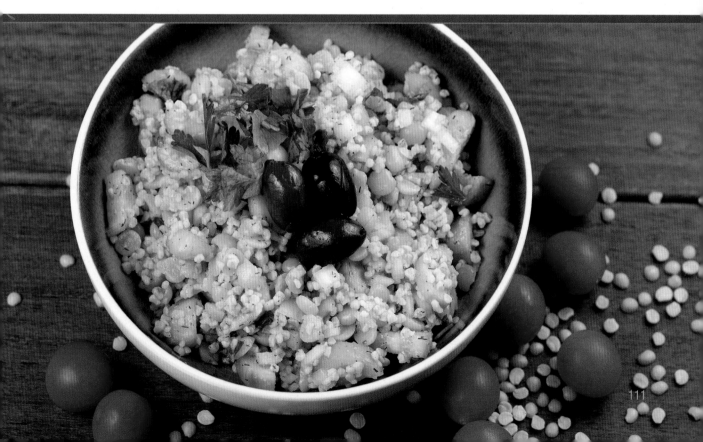

VEGGIE Pad Thai

MAKES 6 SERVINGS

Pad thai is a beloved stir-fried noodle dish. Unfortunately, restaurant versions are often high in sugar, fat, and sodium. In this recipe, marinated tofu and veggies are combined with brown-rice noodles to create a colorful and healthy meal.

1¾ cups **water**

1 cup chopped **fresh cilantro,** lightly packed

3 tablespoons unsweetened **peanut butter**

2 tablespoons **agave nectar**

2 tablespoons freshly squeezed **lemon** or **lime juice**

2 **garlic cloves,** peeled

1 teaspoon grated **fresh ginger**

1½ teaspoons **salt**

1 (14-ounce) package **extra-firm** or **firm tofu,** cut into ½-inch cubes

1 (8-ounce) package brown rice **pad thai noodles**

5 cups chopped **broccoli**

1 cup frozen **corn kernels**

1 cup shredded **carrots**

1 teaspoon **garlic granules**

½ cup finely chopped **scallions,** for garnish

1. To make the marinade, put 1¼ cups of the water in a blender. Add the cilantro, peanut butter, agave nectar, lemon juice, garlic, ginger, and 1 teaspoon of the salt and process until smooth.

2. Put the tofu cubes in a large bowl. Pour all of the marinade on top of the tofu and let marinate in the refrigerator for 8 to 12 hours.

3. Cook the noodles according to the package instructions and set aside.

4. Warm a large, wide nonstick saucepan over medium-high heat for 3 minutes.

5. Lightly mist the surface of the pan with canola oil spray.

6. Use a slotted spoon to remove the tofu from the marinade and put it in the pan in a single layer. Leave behind as much of the marinade as possible (it will be used later for the pad thai sauce). Cook, stirring frequently, until the tofu cubes are golden brown all over, about 8 minutes. Transfer to a clean bowl and set aside. Alternatively, cook the tofu in an air fryer on high until golden brown, about 12 minutes.

7 Lightly mist the pan again with canola oil spray. Add the broccoli, corn, carrots, garlic granules, and ¼ cup of the water and stir with a large spoon. Cover and cook over medium heat, stirring occasionally, until the broccoli is slightly soft, about 7 minutes. If the vegetables start to burn, add the remaining ¼ cup of water.

8 Add the remaining ½ teaspoon salt and the reserved marinade, noodles, and tofu and stir to combine. Cook uncovered until warm, stirring occasionally, about 3 minutes.

9 Garnish with the scallions just before serving.

Stored in an airtight container, the pad thai will keep in the refrigerator for about 4 days.

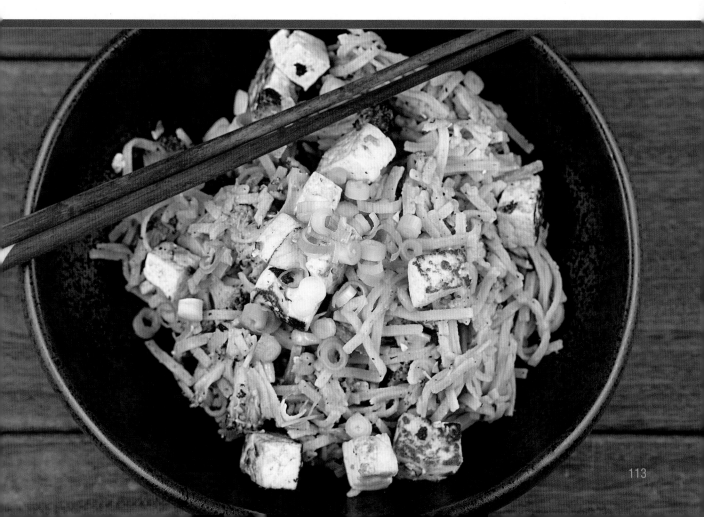

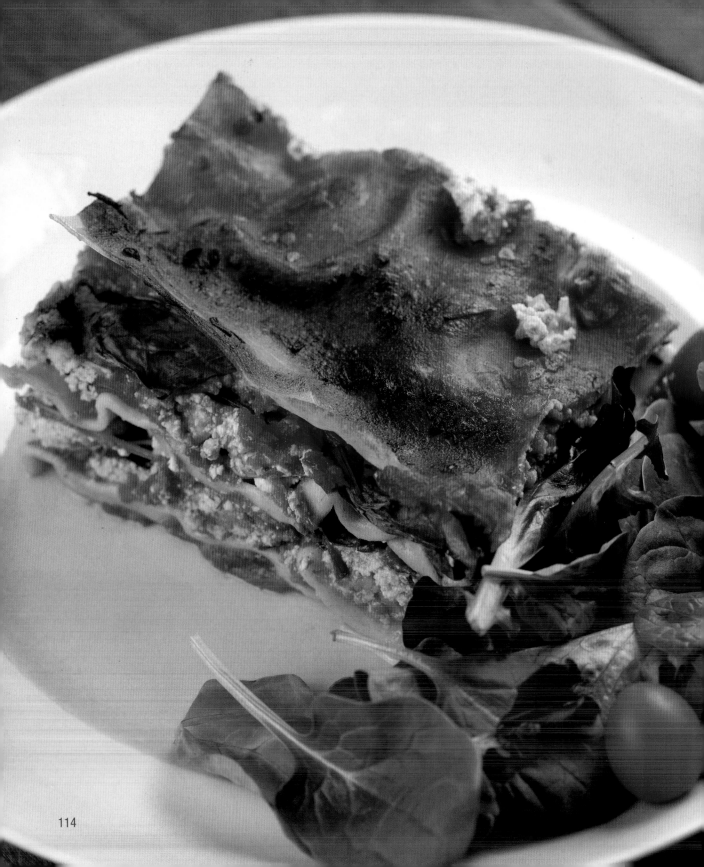

Veggie LASAGNA

MAKES 6 SERVINGS

The surprising partnership of roasted sweet potatoes and tofu makes a spectacular filling for lasagna. Because the noodles aren't cooked in advance, the oven does most of the work for you!

1 large Japanese or regular **sweet potato,** unpeeled

1 (14-ounce) package **extra-firm tofu,** drained

1 (5-ounce) package **baby spinach**

3 tablespoons **Italian seasoning**

½ teaspoon **salt**

6 cups **Marinara Sauce** (page 76) or **Ten-Minute Pasta Sauce** (page 77)

1 (12-ounce) box **whole wheat lasagna noodles**

1. Preheat the oven to 425 degrees F. Line a small baking pan with parchment paper.

2. Lay the sweet potato in the lined pan and bake for 1 hour, until a fork can be easily inserted into the center. Let cool for 20 minutes.

3. Peel and finely chop the sweet potato.

4. Decrease the oven temperature to 350 degrees F.

5. Put the tofu in a large bowl and mash it well with the back of a sturdy fork.

6. Add the sweet potato, spinach, Italian seasoning, and salt and stir until well combined.

7. Pour 1½ cups of the marinara sauce over the bottom of an 8-inch square baking pan.

8. Overlap 5 pieces of the noodles in a single layer on top of the sauce. Spread a layer of the tofu mixture over the noodles. Pour 1½ cups of the marinara sauce evenly over the tofu mixture until it is fully covered.

9. Repeat the steps with another layer of noodles, tofu mixture, and sauce.

10. Add a final layer of noodles and cover with the remaining 1½ cups of sauce.

11. Sprinkle the remaining tofu mixture evenly over the top.

12. Cover the pan with aluminum foil and bake for 45 minutes.

13. Uncover and bake for 15 minutes longer.

Stored in an airtight container in the refrigerator, the lasagna will keep for about 4 days.

CAULIFLOWER Wings

Cauliflower florets are coated with a rich-tasting batter, then cooked in an air fryer (or in the oven) to make these crispy, oil-free, plant-based wings. Dip them in Creamy Cilantro Chutney (page 79), Low-Fat Creamy Salad Dressing (page 80), or ketchup.

1½ cups **rolled oats**

1 cup **chickpea flour**

6 tablespoons **nutritional yeast flakes**

2 teaspoons **smoked paprika**

2 teaspoons **garlic granules**

1 teaspoon **ground ginger**

1 teaspoon **salt**

1 teaspoon **dried oregano**

¾ teaspoon **dried basil**

¾ teaspoon ground **white pepper**

½ teaspoon crushed **red chile flakes**

1½ cups unsweetened plain **soy** or **almond milk**

1½ teaspoons **apple cider vinegar**

1 medium **cauliflower,** cut into 36 florets

1. Put the oats, chickpea flour, nutritional yeast, paprika, garlic granules, ginger, salt, oregano, basil, white pepper, and chile flakes in a large bowl and stir until well combined.

2. Add the milk and vinegar and stir until well incorporated and the batter is smooth.

3. Dip each cauliflower floret into the batter until fully coated.

4. Cook in an air fryer preheated on high. Arrange a single layer of the florets in the basket and cook until crispy, about 10 minutes. Alternatively, preheat the oven to 400 degrees F and line a large baking sheet with parchment paper. Arrange the florets in a single layer on the lined baking sheet and bake for 18 to 20 minutes, until golden brown.

TIP

Stored in an airtight container in the refrigerator, the wings will keep for about 4 days. Warm in a preheated oven at 375 degrees F for about 7 minutes before serving.

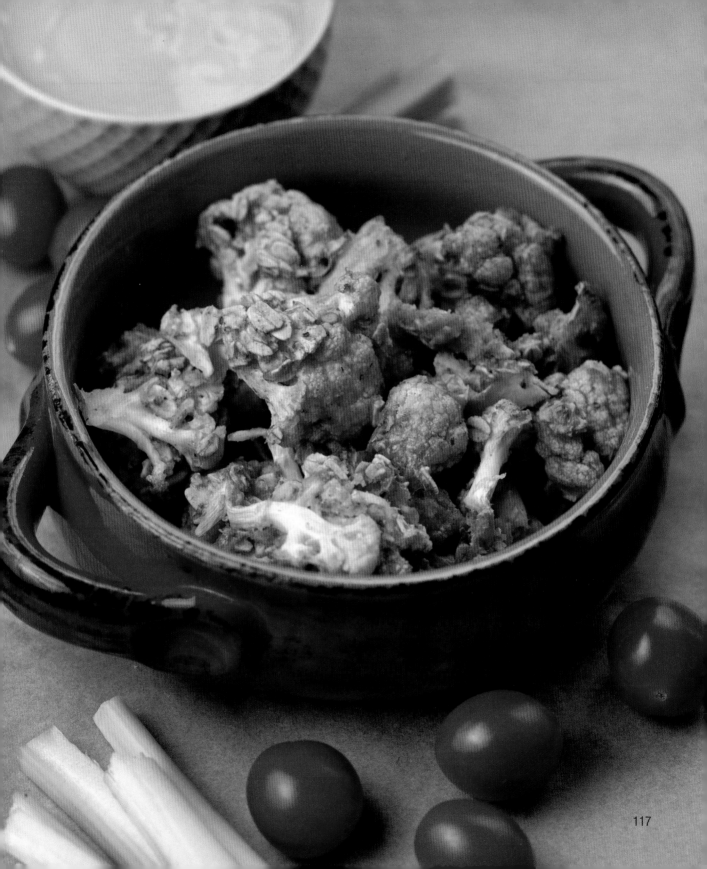

BROWN RICE Vegetable Pilaf

This low-fat, vegan version of a prized North Indian dish harmonizes well with Cucumber Raita (page 83) served alongside it.

1 teaspoon **olive oil**

1 teaspoon **cumin seeds**

1¾ cups frozen **green peas**

1¼ cups shredded or chopped **carrots**

1 teaspoon **ground coriander**

1 teaspoon **salt**

½ teaspoon **ground turmeric**

½ teaspoon **cayenne**

½ teaspoon **garam masala**

1½ cups uncooked brown **basmati rice**

3½ cups **water**

1. Warm the oil in a large saucepan over medium-high heat for 2 minutes.

2. Add the cumin seeds and cook, stirring frequently, until fragrant and golden brown, about 2 minutes. Watch closely so the cumin doesn't burn.

3. Add the peas, carrots, coriander, salt, turmeric, cayenne, and garam masala and cook, stirring frequently, for 4 minutes.

4. Add the rice and water. Stir, cover, and bring to a boil over high heat.

5. Decrease the heat to low and cook covered and undisturbed until the water has been absorbed and the rice is soft, about 35 minutes.

Stored in an airtight container in the refrigerator, the pilaf will keep for about 4 days.

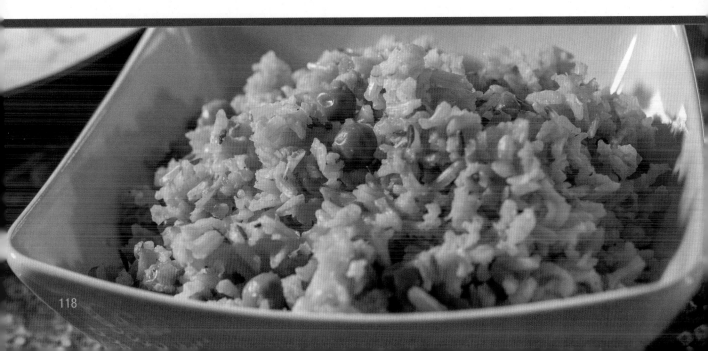

Aloo Gobi (POTATO AND CAULIFLOWER CURRY)

MAKES 6 SERVINGS

For this esteemed dry curry, cauliflower and potatoes are cooked with onions, tomatoes, Indian spices, and herbs. With just a short amount of time and a few seasonings, you'll be impressed that you can make a dish that tastes this complex.

1½ cups finely chopped **onions**

1½ cups finely chopped **tomatoes**

2 teaspoons crushed **garlic**

1 teaspoon grated **fresh ginger**

1 teaspoon **cumin seeds**

1 teaspoon **ground coriander**

1 teaspoon **salt**

½ teaspoon **ground turmeric**

½ teaspoon **cayenne**

¼ teaspoon **garam masala**

1 **cauliflower,** chopped

1½ cups finely chopped unpeeled **potatoes**

½ cup **water,** plus more as needed

1 teaspoon freshly squeezed **lemon** or **lime juice,** plus more as needed

¼ cup finely chopped **fresh cilantro,** lightly packed, for garnish

1 tablespoon finely chopped **green chile,** for garnish

1. Warm a large, wide saucepan over medium-high heat for 3 minutes.

2. Lightly mist the surface of the pan with canola oil spray.

3. Put the onions in the pan and cook, stirring frequently, until golden brown, about 4 minutes.

4. Add the tomatoes, garlic, and ginger and stir until well combined. Cover and cook, stirring frequently, for 4 minutes.

5. Add the cumin seeds, coriander, salt, turmeric, cayenne, and garam masala and stir until well combined. Cover and cook, stirring frequently, for 2 minutes.

6. Add the cauliflower, potatoes, and water and stir to combine. Cover and cook over medium heat, stirring occasionally, until the cauliflower is soft, about 25 minutes. Add more water as needed to prevent burning. Once the cauliflower is soft, increase the heat to evaporate any excess liquid (the curry should be somewhat dry).

7. Stir in the lemon juice, adding more to taste.

8. Garnish with the cilantro and chile just before serving.

Stored in an airtight container, the curry will keep in the refrigerator for about 4 days or in the freezer for about 6 weeks.

Green Beans AND POTATOES

In this sumptuous North Indian classic, green beans and potatoes are rock stars, thanks to a chorus of harmonious spices.

1 teaspoon **canola** or **vegetable oil**

1 teaspoon **cumin seeds**

½ teaspoon **salt**

¼ teaspoon **ground turmeric**

¼ teaspoon **cayenne**

¼ teaspoon **garam masala**

¾ cup **water,** plus more as needed

2 cups chopped fresh or frozen **green beans**

2 cups finely chopped unpeeled **potatoes**

1 Warm the oil in a large, wide nonstick saucepan over medium-high heat for 2 minutes.

2 Add the cumin seeds and cook, stirring frequently, until fragrant and golden brown, about 2 minutes. Watch closely so the cumin doesn't burn.

3 Add the salt, turmeric, cayenne, and garam masala and stir until well combined. Cook, stirring frequently, for 1 minute.

4 Add the water and green beans, cover, and cook, stirring occasionally, for 5 minutes.

5 Add the potatoes and stir until evenly distributed. Cover and cook, stirring occasionally, until the potatoes and green beans are soft, about 15 minutes. Add more water as needed to prevent burning.

TIP

Stored in an airtight container in the refrigerator, the green beans and potatoes will keep for about 4 days.

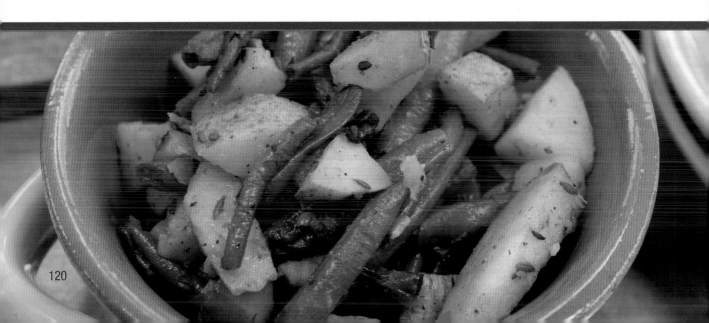

BAKED VEGGIE Pakoras

Pakoras are fritters dipped in chickpea batter and then deep-fried. They are a much-loved Indian snack. For this oil-free version, the pakoras are baked instead of fried, delivering the acclaimed savory taste without the undesirable fat and calories.

2 cups **chickpea flour**

1 teaspoon **ground cumin**

¼ teaspoon **salt**

¼ teaspoon **cayenne**

⅛ teaspoon **garam masala**

1 cup **water**

½ **cauliflower,** chopped

1 unpeeled **potato,** chopped

1 **red onion,** sliced

1. Put the chickpea flour, cumin, salt, cayenne, and garam masala in a large bowl and stir until well combined.

2. To make the batter, add the water and combine using an electric hand or stand mixer until smooth. The batter should be thick.

3. Add the cauliflower, potatoes, and onions and mix with a spoon until the vegetables are fully covered with batter.

4. Cook in an air fryer preheated on high. Arrange a single layer of the pakoras in the basket and cook until crispy, about 10 minutes. Alternatively, preheat the oven to 400 degrees F and line a large baking sheet with parchment paper. Arrange the pakoras in a single layer on the lined baking sheet and bake for 18 to 20 minutes, until golden brown.

Stored in an airtight container in the refrigerator, the pakoras will keep for about 4 days. Reheat in the oven at 375 degrees F for about 7 minutes before serving.

CHICKPEA Crêpes

These savory gluten-free crêpes can be served as a snack or meal. They are fantastic dipped in Creamy Cilantro Chutney (page 79) or ketchup.

1 cup **chickpea flour**

½ teaspoon **salt**

¼ teaspoon **cayenne**

¼ teaspoon **ground turmeric**

¼ teaspoon **garlic granules**

1½ cups **water**

⅓ cup finely chopped **red bell pepper**

⅓ cup finely chopped **red onion**

¼ cup finely chopped **fresh cilantro,** lightly packed

1 Put the chickpea flour, salt, cayenne, turmeric, and garlic granules in a large bowl and stir until well combined.

2 Add the water, bell pepper, onion, and cilantro and combine with a stand or hand mixer to make a smooth batter.

3 Warm a medium nonstick crêpe pan or skillet over medium heat for 3 minutes.

4 Lightly mist the surface of the pan with canola oil spray.

5 Pour ½ cup of the batter into the pan and spread it evenly.

6 Cook over medium heat until the edges of the crêpe are brown, about 4 minutes. Gently flip the crêpe over and cook the other side for 3 to 4 minutes.

Stored in an airtight container in the refrigerator, the batter will keep for about 4 days.

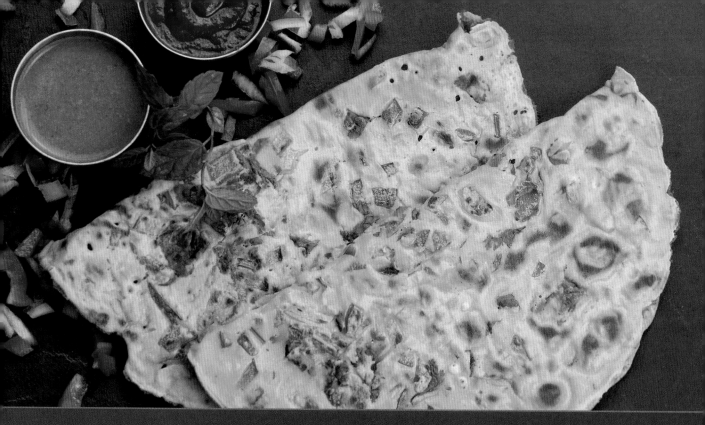

Chickpea Crêpes *(above)*

(below) Black Bean Tacos

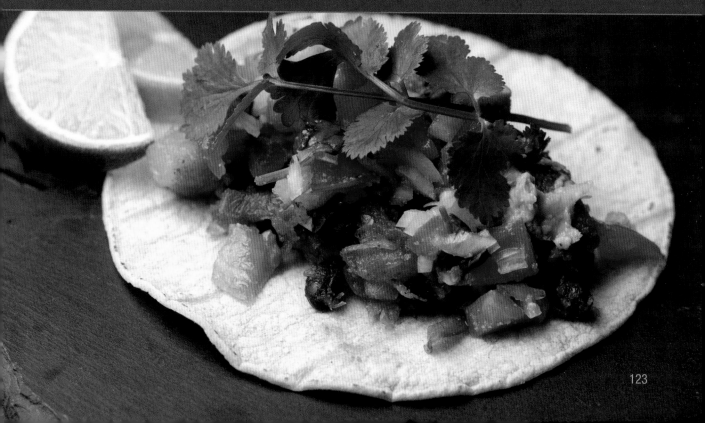

123

BLACK BEAN Tacos

In this fun, easy recipe, seasoned black beans are combined with salsa, guacamole, and shredded lettuce, all piled high on warm corn tortillas.

1 **onion,** thinly sliced

¾ teaspoon **salt**

2 (15-ounce) cans unsalted **black beans,** rinsed and drained

1½ teaspoons **chipotle chile powder**

8 small soft corn **tortillas**

Chopped **lettuce** or **salad greens**

2 cups **Salsa Fresca** (page 45)

1 cup **Classic Guacamole** (page 49)

1. Warm a medium saucepan over medium heat for 3 minutes.

2. Lightly mist the surface of the pan with canola oil spray.

3. Put the onion and salt in the pan and stir to combine. Cook, stirring frequently, until the onion is golden brown, 4 to 5 minutes.

4. Add the beans and chile powder and stir until well combined. Cook, stirring occasionally, until the beans are warm, about 4 minutes.

5. When ready to serve, warm a small skillet over medium heat for 3 minutes.

6. Warm each tortilla in the skillet until golden brown all over, about 2 minutes per side.

7. Serve with lettuce and the beans, salsa, and guacamole.

Stored in an airtight container in the refrigerator, the beans will keep for about 4 days.

Fiesta QUINOA

Quinoa is a whole grain commonly eaten in Latin America. It comes in a variety of colors, all of which are equally nutritious. For this recipe, quinoa is combined with black beans and corn and seasoned with chipotle chile powder. The result? A taste sensation!

1½ cups **quinoa**

3 cups **water**

½ teaspoon **canola, olive, or vegetable oil**

1 (15-ounce) can unsalted **black beans,** rinsed and drained

1 cup frozen **corn kernels**

7 **garlic cloves,** peeled and crushed

2 teaspoons **chipotle chile powder**

¾ teaspoon **salt**

1 cup **Classic Guacamole** (page 49)

Finely chopped **green chiles,** for garnish

1. Warm a large saucepan over medium heat for 3 minutes.

2. Put the quinoa in the pan and roast it, stirring frequently, until it pops and is golden brown, about 5 minutes. (Roasting the quinoa before cooking it imparts a crunchier texture.)

3. Add the water and bring to a boil over high heat. Decrease the heat to low, cover, and cook undisturbed until the water has been absorbed, about 15 minutes. Remove from the heat and fluff with a fork.

4. Put the oil in a large, wide saucepan and warm it over medium heat for 2 minutes.

5. Add the beans, corn, garlic, chile powder, and salt and stir until well combined. Cook, stirring frequently, until heated through, about 5 minutes.

6. Add the quinoa and stir until well combined. Remove from the heat.

7. Dollop ¼ cup of the guacamole on top of or alongside each serving and garnish with the chiles.

Stored in an airtight container in the refrigerator, the quinoa will keep for about 4 days.

Nacho PLATTER

This low-fat, vegan version of nachos, a venerated dish from northern Mexico, is nutritious enough to be the focal point of a meal.

8 ounces (1 cup) dried **black beans,** rinsed, drained, and soaked in water for 8 to 12 hours

1 teaspoon **chipotle chile powder**

½ teaspoon **salt**

8 corn **tortillas**

2 cups **Salsa Fresca** (page 45)

1 cup **Classic Guacamole** (page 49)

Finely chopped **jalapeño chiles,** for garnish

1. Drain and rinse the beans. Put them in a medium saucepan, add enough fresh water to cover the beans completely, and bring to a boil over medium-high heat. Decrease the heat to medium and simmer until soft, 45 to 60 minutes. Add the chile powder and salt to the beans as they boil.

2. If the bean liquid is very thick, add water in ½-cup increments until it has thinned slightly. If the bean liquid is watery, increase the heat and simmer until it has thickened slightly.

3. As the beans are boiling, preheat the oven to 400 degrees F and line a baking sheet with parchment paper.

4. Slice each tortilla into 6 triangles. Place the triangles on the baking sheet in a single layer and bake for 7 to 8 minutes, until lightly browned. Adjust the baking time as needed, depending on your oven and the thickness of the tortillas.

5. Remove the tortilla chips from the oven and let cool on a rack. They will become crispy as they cool.

6. Just before serving, layer the tortilla chips with the beans, salsa, and guacamole. Top with chiles to taste.

Stored in separate airtight containers, the beans will keep in the refrigerator for about 4 days and the chips will keep at room temperature for about 2 days.

Burrito BOWLS

Brown rice and pinto beans are matched with fresh salsa and guacamole in these nourishing, well-balanced bowls.

1½ cups **brown rice**

8 ounces (1 cup) dried **pinto beans,** rinsed, drained, and soaked in water for 8 to 12 hours

1 teaspoon **chipotle chile powder**

½ teaspoon **salt**

2 cups **Salsa Fresca** (page 45)

1 cup **Classic Guacamole** (page 49)

1 Cook the rice on the stove top according to the package instructions or in a rice cooker using the brown rice setting.

2 Drain and rinse the beans. Put them in a medium saucepan, add enough fresh water to cover the beans completely, and bring to a boil over medium-high heat. Decrease the heat to medium and simmer until soft, 45 to 60 minutes. Add the chile powder and salt midway through the cooking cycle.

3 If the sauce is very thick, add water in ½-cup increments until it has thinned slightly. If the sauce is watery, increase the heat and simmer until it has thickened slightly.

4 For each serving, put ½ cup of the rice, ½ cup of the beans, ¼ cup of the salsa, and ¼ cup of the guacamole side by side in a bowl.

Stored in separate airtight containers in the refrigerator, the rice and beans will each keep for about 4 days.

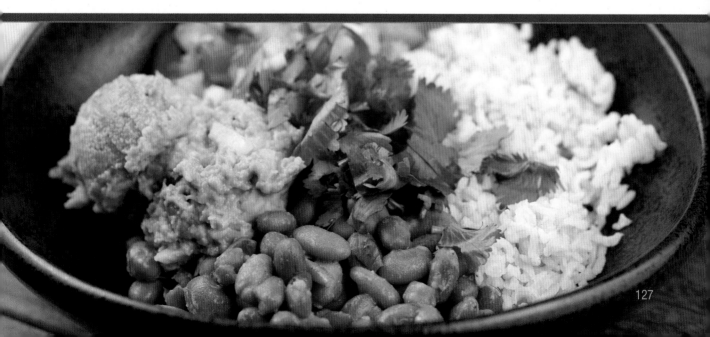

Mexican CASSEROLE

Tortillas, beans, tofu, and homemade salsa share the spotlight in this south-of-the-border layered casserole.

1 (14-ounce) package **extra-firm tofu, drained**

2 (15-ounce) cans unsalted **black beans,** rinsed and drained

2 teaspoons **chipotle chile powder**

½ teaspoon **salt**

12 small corn **tortillas**

6 cups **Restaurant-Style Salsa** (page 79)

1 cup **Classic Guacamole** (page 49)

1 Preheat the oven to 450 degrees F.

2 Crumble the tofu into a large bowl and mash it with the back of a sturdy fork.

3 Add the beans, chile powder, and salt and stir until well combined.

4 Slice each tortilla into 4 pieces.

5 Place a single layer of the tortilla slices in a 9-inch square baking pan. Add a layer of the tofu mixture, then pour a layer of the salsa over it. Repeat with another layer of the tortilla slices, the tofu mixture, and the salsa.

6 Add a final layer of the tortilla slices, followed by a final layer of the remaining salsa. Sprinkle any remaining tofu mixture over the top.

7 Cover the baking pan with foil.

8 Bake covered for 20 minutes, then uncover and bake for 10 minutes longer.

9 Serve hot, with the guacamole on the side.

SPICY Okra

Although okra gets top billing in this time-honored North Indian dish, the spices, in a supporting role, are what really make it a showstopper. To transform it from a side dish into a meal, serve it with whole wheat pita bread and Cucumber Raita (page 83).

½ teaspoon **canola** or **vegetable oil**

1 large **red onion,** chopped

½ teaspoon **cumin seeds**

½ teaspoon **salt**

¼ teaspoon **ground turmeric**

¼ teaspoon **cayenne**

¼ teaspoon **garam masala**

1 (12-ounce) package chopped frozen **okra**

1   Warm the oil in a large nonstick saucepan over medium heat for 2 minutes.

2   Add the onion and cook, stirring frequently, until golden brown, about 4 minutes.

3   Add the cumin seeds, salt, turmeric, cayenne, and garam masala and stir until well combined. Cook, stirring frequently, until the cumin is golden brown, about 2 minutes.

4   Add the okra and stir until well combined. Cook uncovered, stirring frequently, until the okra is soft, about 15 minutes.

Stored in an airtight container in the refrigerator, the okra will keep for about 4 days.

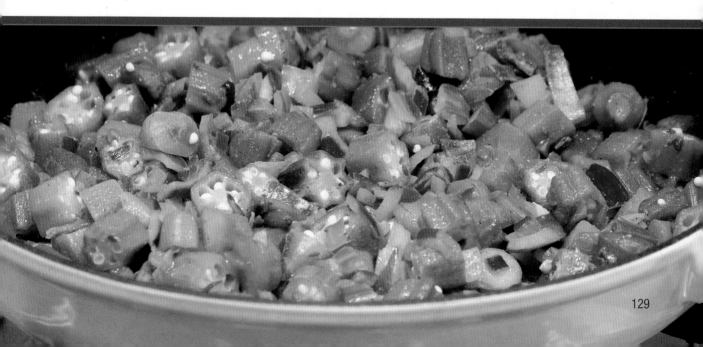

129

Strawberry Ice Cream

CHOCOLATE OR VANILLA Ice Cream

MAKES 4 SERVINGS

Frozen bananas are the foundation of this decadent-tasting, no-added-sugar treat that you can dig into guilt-free for dessert or an afternoon snack.

3 very ripe **bananas,** peeled, broken into chunks, and frozen for at least 8 hours

½ cup unsweetened plain **soy** or **almond milk**

1½ tablespoons unsweetened **cocoa powder,** for chocolate ice cream
(omit for vanilla ice cream)

1 teaspoon **vanilla extract**

1. Put the frozen bananas, milk, cocoa powder (if using), and vanilla extract in a high-speed blender or food processor and process until smooth. If using a regular-speed blender, thaw the frozen bananas for about 5 minutes before processing.

2. Best enjoyed fresh.

Stored in an airtight container in the freezer, the ice cream will keep for about 2 weeks. Warm in the microwave for 15 seconds or let thaw on the counter for about 10 minutes before serving.

Strawberry ICE CREAM

MAKES 4 SERVINGS

Blended frozen strawberries make a compelling snack or a satisfying end-of-meal flourish.

1½ cups chopped fresh **strawberries,** frozen for at least 8 hours

1 cup unsweetened plain **soy** or **almond milk**

2 tablespoons **agave nectar,** plus more as needed

1. Put all the ingredients in a high-speed blender or food processor and process until smooth. If using a regular-speed blender, thaw the frozen strawberries for about 5 minutes before processing. Add more agave nectar to taste, if desired.

2. Best enjoyed fresh.

Stored in an airtight container in the freezer, the ice cream will keep for about 2 weeks. Warm in the microwave for 15 seconds or let thaw on the counter for about 10 minutes before serving.

Chocolate-Cherry ICE CREAM

MAKES 4 SERVINGS

Just a few basic ingredients go into this elegant frozen delight. It tastes so creamy and rich, no one will guess it's actually a health food disguised as dessert.

Stored in an airtight container in the freezer, the ice cream will keep for about 2 weeks. Warm in the microwave for 15 seconds or let thaw on the counter for about 10 minutes before serving.

16 ounces (1 pound) frozen pitted **red cherries**

1 cup unsweetened plain **soy** or **almond milk**

¼ cup **maple syrup**

1½ tablespoons unsweetened **cocoa powder**

1 teaspoon **vanilla extract**

1 Put all the ingredients in a high-speed blender or food processor and process until smooth. If using a regular-speed blender, thaw the frozen cherries for about 5 minutes before processing.

2 Best enjoyed fresh.

MOCHA Smoothie

MAKES 1 SERVING

The union of frozen bananas, cocoa powder, and coffee creates a luxurious, smooth beverage that is sure to please.

½ very ripe **banana**, peeled, broken into chunks, and frozen for at least 8 hours

1 cup unsweetened **soy** or **almond milk**

1½ teaspoons **agave nectar**

1 teaspoon unsweetened **cocoa powder**

1 teaspoon **instant coffee granules**

1 Put all the ingredients in a high-speed blender and process until smooth. If you're using a regular-speed blender, thaw the frozen banana for about 5 minutes before processing.

2 Best enjoyed fresh.

Peanut Butter-CHOCOLATE CHIP COOKIES

MAKES 12 COOKIES

The classic combo of peanut butter and chocolate is front and center in these divine whole-grain cookies.

1 cup **whole wheat pastry flour**

⅔ cup **oat flour**

⅔ cup **sugar**

⅔ cup **vegan chocolate chips**

⅓ cup unsweetened smooth or crunchy **peanut butter**

⅓ cup unsweetened **applesauce**

3 tablespoons **soy milk**

1 teaspoon **vanilla extract**

½ teaspoon **baking soda**

¼ teaspoon **salt**

1. Preheat the oven to 350 degrees F. Line a large baking sheet with parchment paper.

2. Put all the ingredients in a large bowl and combine using an electric hand or stand mixer.

3. Shape into 12 equal cookies. Arrange on the lined baking sheet and bake for about 8 minutes, until golden brown. For a crunchier cookie, bake for 1 to 2 minutes longer.

Stored at room temperature in an airtight container, the cookies will keep for about 4 days.

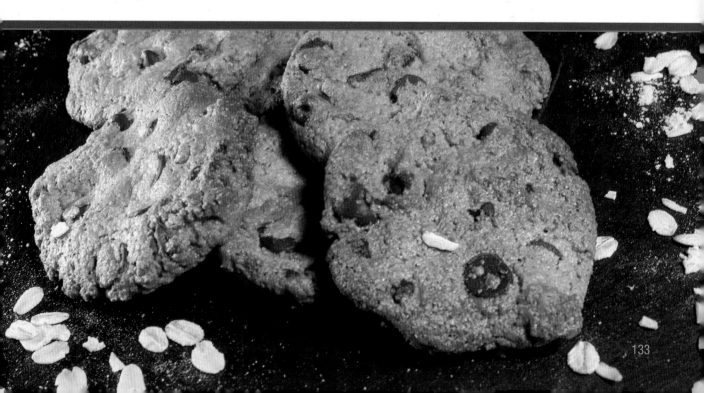

Gingerbread

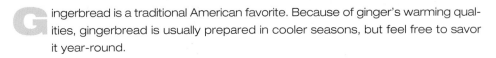ingerbread is a traditional American favorite. Because of ginger's warming qualities, gingerbread is usually prepared in cooler seasons, but feel free to savor it year-round.

2 cups unsweetened plain **soy** or **almond milk**

¼ cup chia seeds or **ground flaxseeds**

¼ cup **molasses**

3 tablespoons **canola** or **vegetable oil**

2 tablespoons **apple cider vinegar**

2 cups **whole wheat pastry flour**

¾ cup **sugar**

1 tablespoon **ground cinnamon**

1 tablespoon **ground ginger**

1¼ teaspoons **baking soda**

1 teaspoon **ground allspice**

⅛ teaspoon **salt**

1. Preheat the oven to 350 degrees F. Line an 8-inch square baking pan with parchment paper.

2. Put the milk, chia seeds, molasses, oil, and vinegar in a large bowl and stir until well combined. Let sit for 10 minutes.

3. Put the pastry flour, sugar, cinnamon, ginger, baking soda, allspice, and salt in a medium bowl and stir until well combined.

4. Add the dry ingredients to the wet ingredients and mix with a hand or stand mixer until well combined.

5. Pour into the lined baking pan and bake for 45 to 50 minutes, until a toothpick inserted in the center comes out clean.

6. Let cool for 10 minutes on a rack before slicing and serving.

Stored in an airtight container in the refrigerator, the gingerbread will keep for 4 to 5 days.

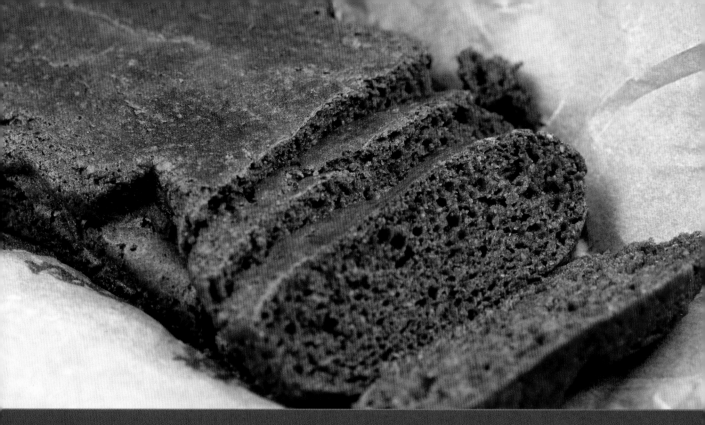

Gingerbread *(above)*

(below) **Chocolate Chip Donuts**

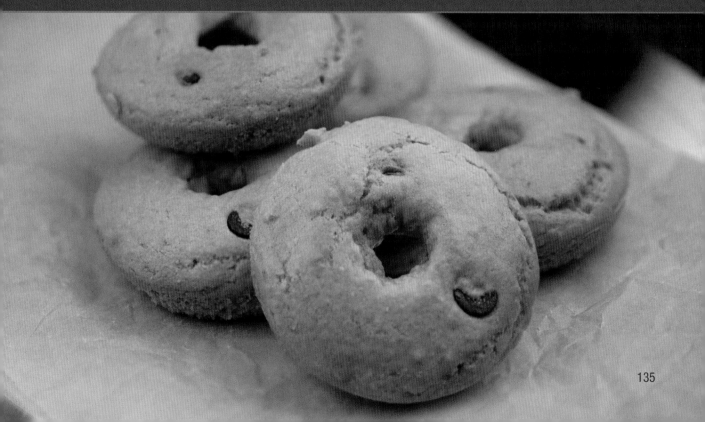

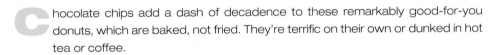

Chocolate Chip DONUTS

Chocolate chips add a dash of decadence to these remarkably good-for-you donuts, which are baked, not fried. They're terrific on their own or dunked in hot tea or coffee.

2¼ cups **whole wheat pastry flour**

⅔ cup **sugar**

½ cup **vegan chocolate chips**

1 teaspoon **baking soda**

1 teaspoon **baking powder**

⅛ teaspoon **salt**

1½ cups unsweetened plain **soy** or **almond milk**

¼ cup **vegetable** or **canola oil**

2 teaspoons **vanilla extract**

1½ teaspoons **apple cider vinegar**

1. Preheat the oven to 350 degrees F. Lightly oil a 12-count donut pan.

2. Put the flour, sugar, chocolate chips, baking soda, baking powder, and salt in a large bowl and stir until well combined.

3. Add the milk, oil, vanilla extract, and vinegar and incorporate using an electric hand or stand mixer until well combined.

4. Portion the batter evenly into the prepared donut pan. Bake for about 15 minutes, until a toothpick inserted in the center of a donut comes out clean.

5. Let cool for 10 minutes before serving.

Let cool completely before storing. Stored in an airtight container in the refrigerator, the donuts will keep for 3 to 4 days.

BLACK BEAN Brownies

t may sound strange to prepare a dessert with black beans, but these gluten-free brownies rival any others when it comes to being luxuriously moist and chocolatey. For a special occasion, top them with Vanilla Ice Cream (page 131).

3 cups unsalted cooked or canned **black beans,** rinsed and drained

¾ cup **water**

⅔ cup **sugar**

½ cup unsweetened **applesauce**

⅓ cup unsweetened **cocoa powder**

¼ cup smooth **almond butter** or **almond flour**

2 tablespoons **ground flaxseeds**

1 teaspoon **baking powder**

1 teaspoon **vanilla extract**

⅛ teaspoon **salt**

1 Preheat the oven to 350 degree F. Line a 12-cup standard muffin pan with cupcake liners.

2 Put all the ingredients in a high-speed blender or food processor and process until smooth. Divide equally among the lined muffin cups.

3 Bake for 25 minutes. Let cool for 30 minutes, then refrigerate for at least 2 hours before serving.

Stored in an airtight container in the refrigerator, the brownies will keep for about 4 days.

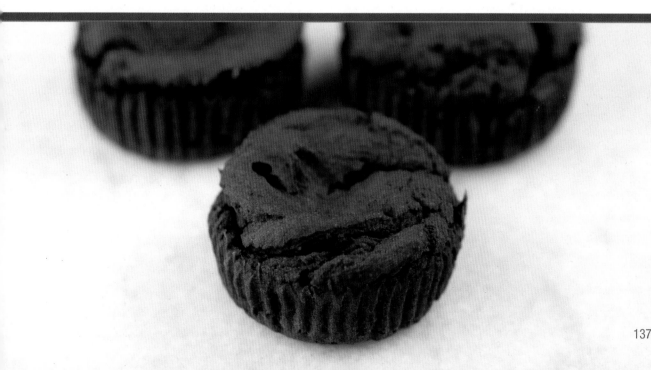

137

Açaí BOWLS

Açaí berries are indigenous to Latin America. For this recipe, the berries' frozen pulp is blended with vegan milk and peanut butter for a frozen treat that is beyond compare.

4 (100-gram) packets frozen **açaí pulp**

1 cup unsweetened plain **soy** or **almond milk**

¼ cup unsweetened smooth **peanut butter**

3 tablespoons **agave nectar**

2 **bananas**, sliced

1 cup **berries** (blackberries, blueberries, or raspberries)

½ cup **Crunchy Granola** (page 21)

Stored in an airtight container in the freezer, the açaí mixture will keep for about 2 weeks. Warm for 15 seconds in the microwave or let thaw on the counter for about 10 minutes before serving.

1 Hold the frozen açaí packets under hot running water for about one minute. Trim the plastic top and pour the pulp into a blender.

2 Add the milk, peanut butter, and agave nectar and process until smooth.

3 Portion the blended mixture into individual bowls. Just before serving, top each bowl with ½ banana, ¼ cup of the berries, and 2 tablespoons of the granola.

Fruit SALAD

What a simple and convenient way to transform fresh fruits into an extra-special dessert! This attractive mix is equally at home at a picnic, on a buffet table, or at a formal dinner party.

4 cups chopped **bananas, apples,** or **pears**

1 cup chopped **mango, watermelon, orange,** or **pineapple**

1 cup fresh **berries**

1 tablespoon **agave nectar**

½ teaspoon freshly squeezed **lemon juice**

¼ teaspoon **salt**

Stored in an airtight container in the refrigerator, the salad will keep for 24 to 36 hours.

1 Put all the ingredients in a large bowl and gently stir to combine.

2 Serve immediately or well chilled.

PINEAPPLE Upside-Down CAKE

MAKES 10 SERVINGS

resh pineapple and whole grains are combined to make a succulent cake that is finger-licking good.

¼ cup plus 2 tablespoons **canola** or **vegetable oil**

1 cup **sugar**

1 **pineapple,** chopped (reserve the juice)

2 cups unsweetened plain **soy** or **almond milk**

1 tablespoon **vinegar** or freshly squeezed **lemon juice**

3 cups **whole wheat pastry flour**

1¼ teaspoons **baking soda**

⅛ teaspoon **salt**

1 teaspoon **vanilla extract**

1 Preheat the oven to 350 degrees F.

2 Oil a 9 x 13-inch baking pan with 2 tablespoons of the oil.

3 Sprinkle ¼ cup of the sugar over the bottom of the pan. Arrange the pineapple evenly over the sugar.

4 Put the milk and vinegar in a small bowl and stir to combine. Let rest for 5 minutes.

5 Put the flour, remaining ¾ cup sugar, and the baking soda and salt in a large bowl. Stir with a dry whisk to combine.

6 Add the milk mixture, remaining ¼ cup oil, the vanilla extract, and ¼ cup of reserved pineapple juice. Stir with a large spoon until smooth and well combined.

7 Pour evenly over the pineapple and bake for 30 minutes.

8 Let cool for at least 20 minutes, then flip the pan over onto a tray to serve.

Stored in an airtight container in the refrigerator, the cake will keep for about 5 days.

Chocolate HUMMUS

If you've never had chocolate hummus, you're in for a delightful surprise. Kids and adults alike will enjoy dipping apple slices in it.

3 (15-ounce) cans unsalted **chickpeas**, rinsed and drained

¾ cup **maple syrup**

½ cup unsweetened **cocoa powder**

½ cup **water,** plus more as needed

⅓ cup **almond flour**

¼ cup plain unsweetened **soy** or **almond milk**

1 teaspoon **vanilla extract**

⅛ teaspoon **salt**

TIP

Stored in an airtight container in the refrigerator, the hummus will keep for about 3 days.

1 Put all the ingredients in a high-speed blender or food processor and process until smooth.

2 Serve immediately or well chilled.

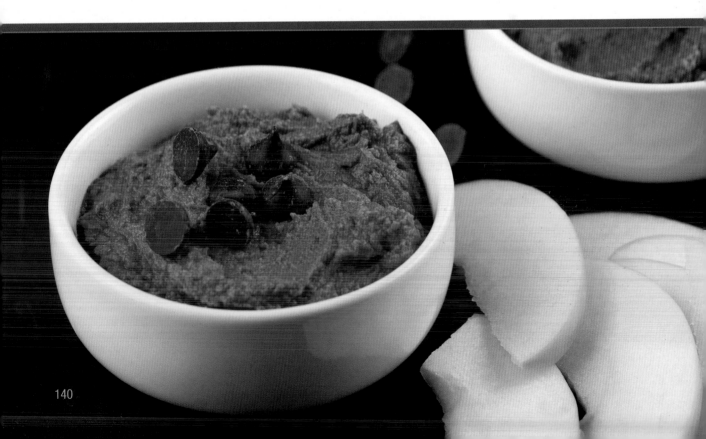

CHICKPEA Blondies

These gluten-free blondies are chock-full of protein. They are so scrumptious, no one will guess their secret ingredient: chickpeas! The chocolate chips impart a rich taste and pleasing crunch.

1½ (15-ounce) cans unsalted **chickpeas,** rinsed and drained

½ cup **almond butter**

⅓ cup **maple syrup**

2 teaspoons **vanilla extract**

¼ teaspoon **salt**

¼ teaspoon **baking powder**

¼ teaspoon **baking soda**

⅓ cup **vegan chocolate chips**

1. Preheat the oven to 350 degrees F. Line an 8-inch square baking pan with parchment paper.

2. Put the chickpeas, almond butter, maple syrup, vanilla extract, salt, baking powder, and baking soda in a large bowl and mix using an electric hand or stand mixer until well combined.

3. Add the chocolate chips and stir until evenly distributed.

4. Pour into the lined baking pan and bake for 25 minutes.

5. Let cool for 20 minutes. Slice into 9 squares and refrigerate for at least 4 hours before serving.

Stored in an airtight container in the refrigerator, the blondies will keep for about 3 days.

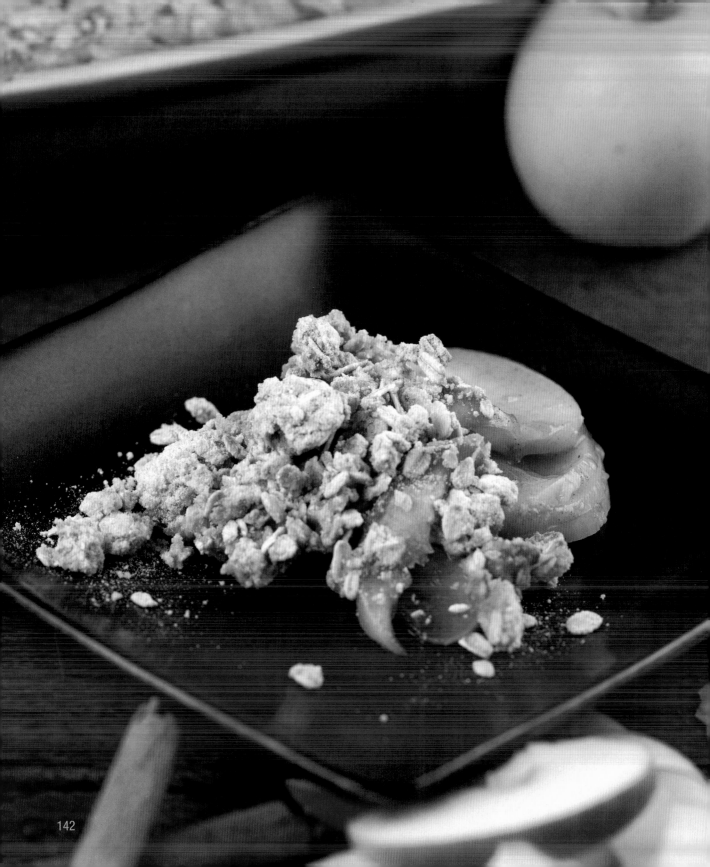

APPLE Crumble

Unlike traditional apple pie, this lightly sweetened crumble is actually good for you! Serve it warm with Vanilla Ice Cream (page 131).

FILLING

6 unpeeled **Honey Crisp apples**, thinly sliced (see tip)

3 tablespoons freshly squeezed **lemon juice**

5 cups **water**

½ cup **cornstarch**

½ cup **brown sugar**

2 teaspoons **ground cinnamon**

½ teaspoon **pumpkin pie spice**

⅛ teaspoon **ground nutmeg**

⅛ teaspoon **salt**

CRUMBLE

1½ cups **rolled oats**

1½ cups **whole wheat pastry flour**

⅓ cup **almond flour**

¼ cup **sugar**

⅛ teaspoon **salt**

½ cup unsweetened plain **soy** or **almond milk**

1. Preheat the oven to 375 degrees F. Line a 13 x 8-inch baking pan with parchment paper.

2. To prepare the filling, put the apple slices in a large bowl and drizzle with the lemon juice. Set aside.

3. Put the water, cornstarch, brown sugar, cinnamon, pumpkin pie spice, nutmeg, and salt in a large saucepan and stir until well combined. Cook over medium heat, stirring frequently, until the mixture comes to a boil, about 8 minutes.

4. Add the apples and stir until well combined. Cover and cook over medium heat, stirring occasionally, for 10 minutes. Remove from the heat and pour into the lined baking pan.

5. To make the crumble, put the oats, pastry flour, almond flour, sugar, and salt in a large bowl and stir until well combined. Slowly stir in the milk until the mixture is crumbly. If the mixture is too wet, add more oats. If the mixture is too dry, add a little more milk.

6. Using your fingers, sprinkle the crumble evenly over the apple filling and bake for 20 minutes.

It is best to avoid peeling the apples because the skin is rich in fiber and other nutrients. Stored in an airtight container in the refrigerator, the crumble will keep for 4 to 5 days. Just before serving, reheat until warm in the microwave or in the oven at 350 degrees F.

References

1. Esselstyn CB Jr. Updating a 12-year experience with arrest and reversal therapy for coronary heart disease (an overdue requiem for palliative cardiology). *Am J Cardiol.* 1999; 84(3): 339–A8. doi:10.1016/s0002-9149(99)00290-8.

2. Esselstyn CB Jr, Gendy G, Doyle J, Golubic M, Roizen MF. A way to reverse CAD? *J Fam Pract.* 2014; 63(7): 356–364b.

3. Esselstyn CB Jr. Resolving the coronary artery disease epidemic through plant-based nutrition. *Prev Cardiol.* 2001; 4(4): 171–177. doi:10.1111/j.1520-037x.2001.00538.x.

4. Ornish D, Scherwitz LW, Billings JH, et al. Intensive lifestyle changes for reversal of coronary heart disease [published correction appears in *JAMA* 1999 Apr. 21; 281(15): 1380]. *JAMA.* 1998; 280(23): 2001–2007. doi:10.1001/jama.280.23.2001.

5. Ornish D, Brown SE, Scherwitz LW, et al. Can lifestyle changes reverse coronary heart disease? The Lifestyle Heart Trial. *Lancet.* 1990; 336(8708): 129–133. doi:10.1016/0140-6736(90)91656-u.

6. Lee YM, Kim SA, Lee IK, et al. Effect of a brown rice based vegan diet and conventional diabetic diet on glycemic control of patients with type 2 diabetes: a 12-week randomized clinical trial. *PLoS One.* 2016; 11(6): e0155918. Published 2016 Jun 2. doi:10.1371/journal.pone.0155918.

7. Tonstad S, Butler T, Yan R, Fraser GE. Type of vegetarian diet, body weight, and prevalence of type 2 diabetes. *Diabetes Care.* 2009; 32(5): 791–796. doi:10.2337/dc08-1886.

8. Orlich MJ, Fraser GE. Vegetarian diets in the Adventist Health Study 2: a review of initial published findings. *Am J Clin Nutr.* 2014; 100 Suppl 1(1): 353S–8S. doi:10.3945/ajcn.113.071233.

9. Satija A, Bhupathiraju SN, Rimm EB, et al. Plant-based dietary patterns and incidence of type 2 diabetes in US men and women: results from three prospective cohort studies. *PLoS Med.* 2016; 13(6): e1002039. Published 2016 Jun 14. doi:10.1371/journal.pmed.1002039.

10. Wright N, Wilson L, Smith M, Duncan B, McHugh P. The BROAD study: a randomised controlled trial using a whole food plant-based diet in the community for obesity, ischaemic heart disease or diabetes. *Nutr Diabetes.* 2017; 7(3): e256. Published 2017 Mar 20. doi:10.1038/nutd.2017.3.

11. Barnard ND, Cohen J, Jenkins DJ, Turner-McGrievy G, Gloede L, Jaster B, Seidl K, Green AA, Talpers S. A low-fat vegan diet improves glycemic control and cardiovascular risk factors in a randomized clinical trial in individuals with type 2 diabetes. *Diabetes Care*. 2006 Aug; 29(8): 1777–1783. doi:10.2337/dc06-0606. PMID: 16873779.

12. Heart Disease Facts. Centers for Disease Control and Prevention website. https://www.cdc.gov/heartdisease/facts.htm. Updated September 8, 2020. Accessed October 29, 2020.

13. Cardiovascular Diseases. World Health Organization website. https://www.who.int/news-room/fact-sheets/detail/cardiovascular-diseases-(cvds). Updated May 17, 2017. Accessed October 29, 2020.

14. Devries S, Willett W, Bonow RO. Nutrition education in medical school, residency training, and practice. *JAMA*. 2019; 321(14): 1351–1352. doi:10.1001/jama.2019.1581.

15. What's at stake in nutrition education during med school. American Medical Association website. https://www.ama-assn.org/education/accelerating-change-medical-education/whats-stake-nutrition-education-during-med-school. Updated July 13, 2015. Accessed October 29, 2020.

16. Omega-3 fatty acids. National Institutes of Health website. https://ods.od.nih.gov/factsheets/Omega3FattyAcids-HealthProfessional. Updated October 1, 2020. Accessed January 15, 2021.

17. Rehm CD, Peñalvo JL, Afshin A, Mozaffarian D. Dietary intake among US adults, 1999–2012. *JAMA*. 2016; 315(23): 2542–2553. doi:10.1001/jama.2016.7491.

18. Micha R, Peñalvo JL, Cudhea F, Imamura F, Rehm CD, Mozaffarian D. Association between dietary factors and mortality from heart disease, stroke, and type 2 diabetes in the United States. *JAMA*. 2017; 317(9): 912–924. doi:10.1001/jama.2017.0947.

Index

Page references for sidebars and recipe names appear in italics.

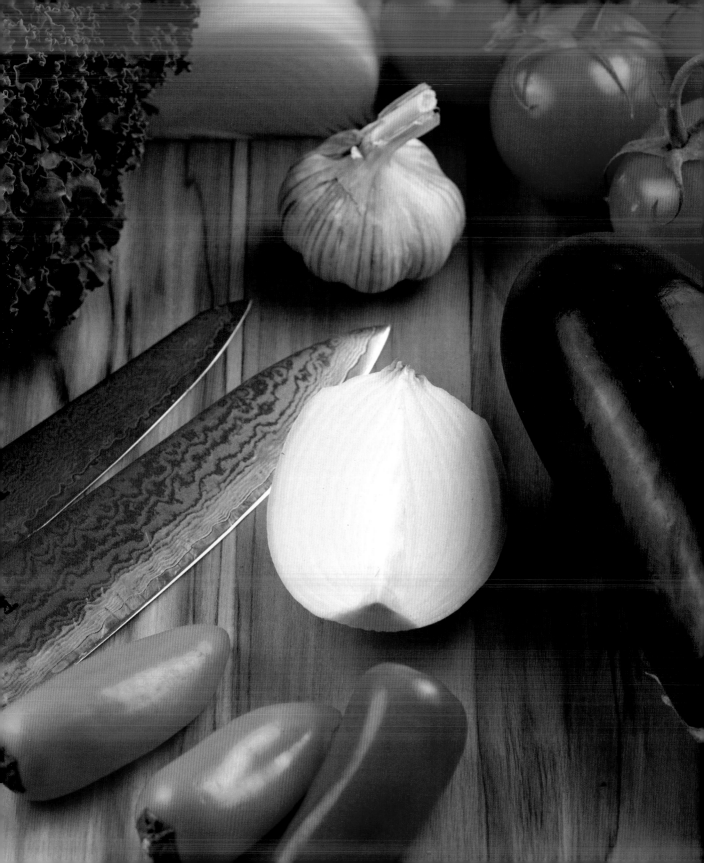

About the Author

Dr. Vanita Rahman, MD, is a board-certified physician in internal medicine. She spent more than fifteen years practicing internal medicine with Kaiser Permanente, where she launched a very popular and successful plant-based weight-loss program. Currently, Dr. Rahman is the clinic director at the Barnard Medical Center and the Physicians Committee for Responsible Medicine, where she leads clinical research, conducts nutrition education programs, and provides patient care with an emphasis on plant-based nutrition. She is also a clinical instructor in medicine at the George Washington University School of Medicine and frequently speaks at international conferences about the role of nutrition in chronic disease.

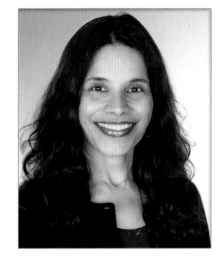

In addition, Dr. Rahman is a certified nutritionist and personal trainer. She has authored several books on plant-based nutrition as well as articles that have been published in peer-reviewed medical journals. In her free time, Dr. Rahman enjoys spending time with family and friends, traveling, exercising, and experimenting with new recipes.

@Dr.Vanita.Rahman (Instagram)

@DocVanita (Twitter)

Dr. Vanita Rahman (Facebook)

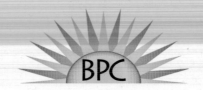

books that educate, inspire, and empower

To find your favorite books on plant-based cooking and nutrition,
raw-foods cuisine, and healthy living, visit:

BookPubCo.com

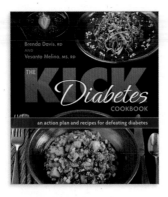

The Kick Diabetes Cookbook
An Action Plan and Recipes
for Defeating Diabetes
Brenda Davis, RD & Vesanto Melina, MS, RD
978-1-57067-359-7 • $19.95

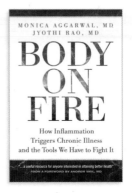

Body On Fire
How Inflammation Triggers Chronic Illness
and the Tools We Have to Fight It
Monica Aggarwal, MD & Jyothi Rao, MD
978-1-57067-392-4 • $17.95

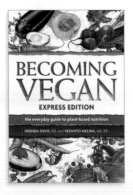

Becoming Vegan Express Edition
The Everyday Guide to Plant-Based Nutrition
Brenda Davis, RD & Vesanto Melina, MS, RD
978-1-57067-295-8 • $22.95

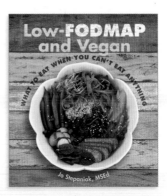

Low-FODMAP and Vegan
What to Eat When You Can't Eat Anything
Jo Stepaniak, MSEd
978-1-57067-337-5 • $19.95

Purchase these titles from your favorite book source or buy them directly from:
BPC • PO Box 99 • Summertown, TN 38483 • 1-888-260-8458

Free shipping and handling on all orders